普通高等教育"十一五"国家级规划教材　配套教学用书
新世纪（第二版）全国高等中医药院校规划教材

State Textbook for General Higher Education in the "11th 5-Year Plan"
"New Century" (2nd Edition) State Textbook for Higher Education
in Chinese Medicine

Student Companion Book

中医舌诊彩色图谱

（中英文对照）

Chromatic Illustrated Atlas of Tongue Diagnosis in Chinese Medicine

（Chinese-English）

主　　编（Chief Editor）	龚一萍 Gong Yiping
副 主 编（Vice Chief Editor）	徐　珊 Xu Shan
	柴可夫 Chai Kefu
编　　委（Members）	倪美文 Ni Meiwen
	陈素珍 Chen Suzhen
	祝春燕 Zhu Chunyan
主　　审（Chief Examine）	范永升 Fan Yongsheng
英文翻译（Translator）	Alice Huynh
	龚一萍 Gong Yiping

中国中医药出版社
·北　京·

图书在版编目（CIP）数据

中医舌诊彩色图谱：中英文对照/龚一萍主编. —2 版. —北京：中国中医药出版社，2010.2（2011.8 重印）

ISBN 978-7-80231-839-7

Ⅰ.①中… Ⅱ.①龚… Ⅲ.①舌诊—图谱—中医学院—教学参考资料—汉、英 Ⅳ.①R241.25-64

中国版本图书馆 CIP 数据核字（2009）第 233647 号

中 国 中 医 药 出 版 社 出 版
北京市朝阳区北三环东路 28 号易亨大厦 16 层
邮政编码 100013
传真 010 64405750
北京市松源印刷有限责任公司印刷
各地新华书店经销
*
开本 850×1168 1/16 印张 8.25 字数 390 千字
2006 年 4 月第 1 版 2011 年 8 月第 2 版第 2 次印刷
书 号 ISBN 978-7-80231-839-7
*
定价 35.00 元
网址 www.cptcm.com

前 言

　　舌诊是中医的特色诊法之一，是医生诊病的重要依据。因此舌诊教学内容既要重视中医舌诊的基本理论、基本知识的传授，更要注意培养学生望舌的基本技能。

　　《中医舌诊彩色图谱（中英文对照）》根据舌诊教学的特点及教学需要，以最新教学大纲为依据和主线，紧扣舌诊的主要知识点编写。介绍知识点包括：舌象特征、临床意义、英文翻译、舌象图片4部分。舌象图片中除了反映相应知识点——舌象的特征外，还选取了所拍舌象病人的相关信息，有利于病证结合学习。文字内容为中英文对照，适用于中外学生使用。本书特色：①配套教材，按知识点介绍，脉络清楚。②每一知识点后均有对应的舌象图片，为学生学习舌象构建了很好的直观形象。全书共收图片200幅左右，均是近3年来作者从临床拍摄的最新舌象图片。③中英文对照版本，面对国内外学习中医的学生，有利于中医文化的对外交流。读者对象为在校学生、留学生、成人教育函授学生、一般读者。

　　本书在启动、编写与审阅过程中，中国中医药出版社的有关同志给予了大力支持；在舌象收集的过程中，浙江中医药大学第一附属医院、浙江中医药大学第二附属医院、杭州市中医院、杭州市红会医院相关科室和部门及医生给予了很大帮助，在此一并致谢。

　　舌象图谱化、中英文对照的编写是一项有利于中医教育的工作，编写者虽然身在教学临床一线，但编写这类图书是一项创新性的工作，因此书中缺点和错误在所难免，敬请读者指正。

龚一萍

2009 年 12 月

Foreword

Tongue diagnosis is a distinguishing feature of TCM diagnostic methods, and an important foundation for physicians in diagnosing diseases. Therefore, the content for teaching and learning tongue diagnosis not only places importance on the theoretical foundation of TCM and basic know-ledge of skills, but also focuses on fostering students' basic abilities in observing tongues.

Chromatic Illustrated Atlas of Tongue Diagnosis in Chinese Medicine (Chinese-English), based on the up-to-date teaching programme, is a compilation for helping grasp the essential points for teaching and learning tongue diagnosis. The essential points cover four aspects: the characteristics for tongue manifestations, its clinical significance, English translation, and photographs of tongue manifestations. Not only do the photographs reflect the characteristics of the corresponding essential points, but there is a collection of more relevant data from those patients whose photographs of tongue manifestations were taken, beneficial to the study of diseases and their patterns. This book is written in Chinese-English bilingual form, suitable for both Chinese and foreign students. The special features of this book are: ① A complete set of teaching material, attached to the state-planned text-books, is presented according to the essential points, and with a clear sequence. ② At the conclusion of every essential point, there is a photograph of the corresponding tongue manifestation, giving learners a very good visual image. Approximately 200 photographs in the book are collected and photographed by the author from the clinic in the last 3 years, making them the up-to-date photographs of tongue manifestations. ③ A Chinese-English bilingual edition is compiled for Chinese and Foreign students studying Chinese Medicine, helping promote the cultural exchange of Chinese Medicine with foreign countries. The target audience is general readers, such as local students, foreign students, and adults studying by correspondence.

At the commencement of writing this book, through the process of compilation and critical examination, relevant staffs at the China Press of Traditional Chinese Medicine have given their immense support; in the course of collecting tongue manifestations, the administrations, faculties and doctors in The First and Second Affiliated Hospital of Zhejiang Chinese Medical University, Hangzhou City Hospital of TCM, Hangzhou City Honghui Hospital have been of great help. Their support and help are greatly appreciated with deep thanks.

The collection of illustrative photographs, compilation of the Chinese-English bilingual book is a valuable asset for the teaching of Chinese Medicine. Although the author has been working in teaching and clinic for years, it is a innovative work to compile this kind of books and the deficiencies and errors may occur. The author is looking forward earnestly to the readers' corrections and suggestions.

Gong Yiping
December, 2009

目 录
CONTENT

目　　录

CONTENT

中医舌诊彩色图谱
（中英文对照）

Chromatic Illustrated Atlas of Tongue Diagnosis in Chinese Medicine
（Chinese-English）

第一章

舌 诊 概 说

　　舌诊是通过观察舌质和舌苔的变化，了解机体生理功能和病理情况的诊察方法，是望诊的重要内容，是中医诊法的特色之一。舌诊具有悠久的历史，早在《黄帝内经》中就有关于望舌诊病的记载，如《素问·刺热》曰："肺热病者，先渐然厥，起毫毛，恶风寒，舌上黄。"指出表邪传里，肺胃热盛，舌苔变黄的转化规律。汉·张仲景《伤寒杂病论》将舌诊作为中医辨证论治法则的一个组成部分。在《金匮要略·惊悸吐衄下血胸满瘀血病脉证治》中指出："病人胸满，唇痿舌青……为有瘀血。"以舌青作为有瘀血的依据。元代舌诊专著《敖氏伤寒金镜录》问世，载舌象图36幅，结合临床，进行病机分析，并确定方药及推测预后。明清时代温病学派兴起，对辨舌验齿尤为重视，在研究温热病的过程中，总结出一套"温病察舌"的方法，对温病的辨证论治起到重要的指导作用。由于舌与脏腑气血津液关系十分密切，其变化与体内的各种变化同步，所以舌象是反映人体的非常灵敏的标尺，也可以说舌象是窥测内脏变化的"窗口"，也有人比作反映内脏变化的"镜子"。临床实践证明，凡体质禀赋的强弱、正气的盛衰、病情的浅深、预后的好坏均能客观地从舌象上反映出来，为医生临床诊断提供重要依据。

　　近代，随着医学科学的发展，对舌诊的研究更加深入，开展了舌诊现代化、客观化的研究，对舌象形成的原理有了更加深入的了解，对舌象的临床应用有了新的拓宽和发展。

CHAPTER ONE

AN OVERVIEW OF TONGUE DIAGNOSIS

Tongue diagnosis is accomplished primarily by assessing the changes in the proper and tongue coating. It is a diagnostic tool that helps to understand the mechanisms of the body's physiology as well as pathology of diseases. It is an important part of observation diagnosis as well as being a unique feature of TCM diagnostic methods. Tongue diagnosis has had a very long history, documentation of tongue diagnosis for diseases started as early as the *Yellow Emperor's Internal Classic* (*Huang Di Nei Jing*) of the Warring States Period. For example, from the chapter *Plain Questions • Acupuncture in the Treatment of Febrile Disease*, "In febrile diseases of the Lungs, the patient will have sudden chills and goose bumps, aversion to wind and cold, yellow coating on the tongue." identifying the transformation pattern of tongue coating to a yellow color in correspondence to an external pathogen transferring internally, leading to exuberant heat in the Lungs and Stomach. In the Han Dynasty, Zhang Zhongjing utilized tongue diagnosis as part of his Selecting Treatment by Differentiating Syndromes (STDS) process as prescribed in his compilation the *Treatise on Cold-induced and Miscellaneous Diseases* (*Shang Han Za Bing Lun*). The *Synopsis of the Golden Chamber • On Pulse Syndrome Complex and Treatment of Convulsions and Palpitations*, *Hematemesis*, *Hematochezia*, *Chest Fullness and Blood Stasis*. states: "Patient with fullness in the chest, flaccid lips and blue tongue, ··· indicating there is blood stasis." As a result, a blue tongue is the basic sign of blood stasis. The Yuan Dynasty saw the first text devoted to Tongue Diagnosis published: The *Ao's Record of the Golden Mirror of Cold-induced Disorders*, containing 36 illustrations, each accompanied by an explanatory on the clinical pathogenesis, as well as herbal treatment and the conjecture of a prognosis. During the Ming and Qing Dynasties arose the School of Febrile Diseases, which placed great significance on tongue differentiating and inspection of the teeth. Through the process of researching febrile diseases came the formation of the technique "Observing the Tongue to Identify Febrile Disease", hence providing essential guidance to the differential diagnosis of febrile diseases. Given the close relationship between the tongue and the Qi, Blood, and Body Fluids of the ZangFu, changes of the tongue and changes within the body occur simultaneously, thus the manifestation of the tongue is an extremely sensitive gauge of a patient's condition. It can also be said that the form of the tongue is a "window" to peek at changes of the internal organs, or that the tongue is a "mirror" that reflects on the changes of the internal organs. Through clinical experiences, it is proven that observing the form of the tongue provides an objective reflection of the strength of a body's inherited constitution, the prosperity or decline of the anti-pathogenic Qi, the severity of a disease, a good or poor prognosis, hence it is a basic yet vital diagnostic tool for a TCM practitioner to utilize in practice.

Through the development of modern medical science, the research of tongue diagnosis has become more in-depth, launching its modernization, offering objective researches, providing a better and more thorough understanding of the principle of tongue diagnosis, broadening and providing further development for the clinical use of tongue diagnosis.

第一节 舌的形态结构

舌为一肌性器官，由黏膜和舌肌组成，它附着于口腔底部、下颌骨、舌骨，呈扁平而长形。其主要功能与味觉、发音、搅拌食物、协助吞咽有关。

舌体的上面称舌背，下面称舌底。舌背又分为舌体与舌根两部分（图1-1）。伸舌时一般只能看到舌体，故中医诊舌的部位主要是舌体。

中医学将舌体的前端称为舌尖；舌体的中部称为舌中；舌体的后部、人字形界沟之前称为舌根；舌两边称为舌边（图1-2）。

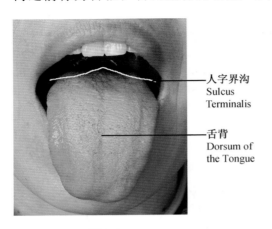

图 1-1

人字界沟
Sulcus Terminalis

舌背
Dorsum of the Tongue

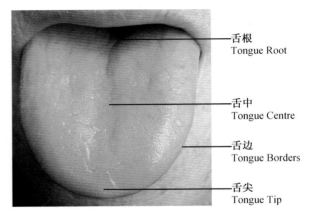

图 1-2

舌根
Tongue Root

舌中
Tongue Centre

舌边
Tongue Borders

舌尖
Tongue Tip

舌体的正中有一条纵形沟纹，称为舌正中沟（图1-3）。

当舌上卷时，可看到舌底。舌底正中有一纵行皱褶，称为舌系带（图1-4）。

舌系带终点两侧各有一个小圆形突起，叫舌下肉阜，有腺管开口于此，中医称其左侧的为金津，右侧的为玉液，是胃津、肾液上潮的孔道。

舌面覆盖一层半透明的黏膜，黏膜皱折成许多细小突起，称为舌乳头。

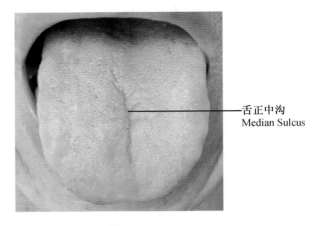

图 1-3

舌正中沟
Median Sulcus

根据舌乳头形态不同，分为丝状乳头、蕈状乳头、轮廓乳头和叶状乳头4种，其中丝状乳头与蕈状乳头与舌象形成有着密切关系，轮廓乳头、叶状乳头与味觉有关。

SECTION ONE   THE FORM AND STRUCTURE OF THE TONGUE

The tongue is a muscular organ occupying the floor of the oral cavity. It is composed of a mucous membrane and tongue muscles and is attached to the hyoid bone and the mandible, appearing as a flat and elongated profile. It is the primary organ of taste, important in the formation of speech, and manipulating food for chewing and swallowing.

The topside of the tongue is called the dorsum of the tongue, and the underside is called the bottom of the tongue. The dorsum of the tongue can be divided into two parts, the tongue body and the tongue root (Diagram 1-1). On extending the tongue, typically only the tongue body is seen. Thus the most significant component in TCM tongue diagnosis is the tongue body.

The front of the tongue body is called the tip of the tongue; The central part of the tongue body is labeled the middle of the tongue; The rear part of the tongue body, in front of the V-shaped groove (sulcus terminalis) is the root of the tongue; The two sides of the tongue body are the tongue borders (Diagram 1-2).

Down the center of the tongue body is a vertical groove, called the median sulcus (Diagram 1-3).

When the tongue is turned upwards, the underside of the tongue is visible. In the middle line, it is elevated into a distinct vertical fold, called the frenulum linguae (Diagram 1-4).

On either side at the base of the frenulum linguae are two spherical protrusions called the sublingual papillae, the duct for the submandibular gland (Wharton's duct) opens into this papillae, in TCM the left side is called Jinjin (acupoint name), and the right side the Yuye (acupoint name); these are the upper passage ways for the body fluids of the Stomach and Kidneys respectively.

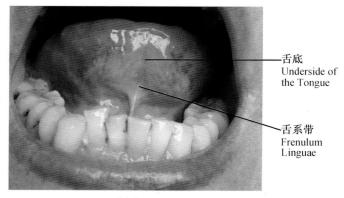

舌底
Underside of
the Tongue

舌系带
Frenulum
Linguae

图 1-4

The surface of the tongue is covered by a semi-transparent mucous membrane, the upper surface is covered with small projections called papillae. Due to the variation in shapes of these papillae they are further categorized into four groups: the filiform, fungiform, foliate, and vallate. Among the four, filiform and fungiform are the papillae primarily associated with the appearance or manifestation of the tongue in TCM. The foliate and vallate papillae are more closely related to the sense of taste.

丝状乳头数目最多，分布在整个舌面，呈圆锥状，高约 0.5～2.5mm，呈角化树状。脱落细胞、食物残渣、细菌、黏液等填充其间隙，形成白色苔状物，称为舌苔。

蕈状乳头数目较少，上部圆钝如球，根部细小形成蕈状。蕈状乳头主要分布在舌尖和舌边，其余散布于丝状乳头之间，乳头表面的上皮细胞透明，透过上皮隐约可见乳头内的毛细血管，肉眼所见如一个小红点。蕈状乳头的形态、色泽改变，是舌质变化的主要因素。

第二节　舌诊的原理和意义

舌与脏腑、经络、气血津液有着密切的联系，主要通过经络和经筋联系起来。

一、舌与脏腑经络的关系

舌为心之苗，手少阴心经之别系舌本。通过望舌色，可以了解人体气血运行情况，从而反映"心主血脉"的功能。此外，舌体运动是否灵活自如，语言是否清晰，在一定程度上又能反映"心藏神"的功能。《灵枢·脉度》还指出："心气通于舌，心和则舌能知五味矣。"说明舌的味觉与心神的功能亦有关。

舌为脾之外候，足太阴脾经连舌本、散舌下。舌居口中，司味觉，《灵枢·脉度》说："脾气通于口，脾和则口能知五谷矣。"故中医有脾开窍于口之说。中医学还认为，舌苔是由胃气蒸化谷气上承于舌面而成的，与脾胃运化功能相应；舌体赖气血充养。所以舌象是全身营养和代谢功能的反映，与脾主运化、化生气血的功能直接有关。

The number of filiform papillae is the greatest of the four; it is distributed all over the tongue. It appears as a conical shape, its approximate height is $0.5 \sim 2.5$mm, projecting from their apices are numerous filamentous processes, epithelium of which they are composed, which has here undergone a peculiar modification, the cells having become carnified and elongated into dense, imbricated, brush-like processes. Epithelial cells, food remnants, bacteria, mucous etc fill up the intervals generating a whitish fur-like substance, which is called the tongue coating.

The number of fungiform papillae in comparison is fewer than that of the filiform papillae, they are broad and rounded at their extremities yet narrow at their attachment to the tongue, hence it is named fungiform. It is found chiefly at the sides and apex of the tongue, and interspersed between the filiform papillae. The surface of the fungiform papillae is covered with a transparent membrane that makes it possible to see the blood capillaries lying just beneath it, giving off a red color, and appearing as red spots to the naked eye. The change in form and color of the fungiform papillae is the main cause of changes that happen to the tongue proper or tongue substance.

SECTION TWO   THE SIGNIFICANCE AND PRINCIPLE OF TONGUE DIAGNOSIS

The tongue has close relationships with the internal organs, meridians, Qi, Blood and Body Fluids through its connections with the channels and the muscles along the channels.

1. The Relationship Between the Tongue, and the Internal Organs, Meridians

The tongue is the sprout of the Heart. Collateral of the Hand Shao Yin Heart Meridian flows to the root of the tongue. Examining the tongue can help to understand the movement of Qi and Blood within the body, thus it can reflect on the condition of the function where "Heart Governs the Blood vessels". Apart from this, the agility of the tongue, the clarity of speech can also reflect on the function where the "Heart houses the Mind". *Spiritual Pivot • Degree of Pulse* points out: "Heart Qi leads to the Tongue, if Heart is in harmony the tongue can distinguish the five tastes." This establishes that there is an intimate relationship between the tongue's sense of taste and the function of the Heart's Mind.

The tongue is the external manifestation of the Spleen, foot Tai Yin Spleen Meridian connects to the root of the tongue and disperses under the tongue. The tongue is situated within the mouth, and has the ability to taste. *Spiritual Pivot • Degree of Pulse* states: "Spleen Qi leads to the mouth, if Spleen is in harmony the mouth can taste the five grains." Thus in TCM the Spleen opens into the mouth. TCM also holds that the tongue coating is a result of Stomach Qi steaming and transporting food essences that rises to the surface of the tongue as a by-product, corresponding to the Spleen and Stomach's functions of transformation and transportation; the tongue relies on the nourishment from Qi and Blood. Therefore the form of the tongue, manifesting the whole body's state of nourishment and metabolism, has direct connection with the Spleen's functions of transportation and transformation, and the production of Qi and Blood.

肾藏精，足少阴肾经夹舌本；肝藏血、主筋，其经脉络于舌本；肺系上达咽喉，与舌根相连。其他脏腑组织，通过经络直接或间接同舌产生联系，从而使舌成为反映机体功能状况的镜子。一旦体内发生病变，就会出现舌象变化，所以观察舌象的各种变化，可以测知体内脏腑的病变。

脏腑病变反映于舌面，具有一定的分布规律。根据历代医籍记载，其中比较一致的说法是：舌质候五脏病变，侧重血分；舌苔候六腑病变，侧重气分。舌尖多反映上焦心肺病变；舌中部多反映中焦脾胃病变；舌根部多反映下焦肾的病变；舌两侧多反映肝胆的病变（图1-5）。

此外，《伤寒指掌·察舌辨证法》还有"舌尖属上脘，舌中属中脘，舌根属下脘"的说法。据临床观察，如心火上炎多出现舌尖红赤或破碎；肝胆气滞血瘀常见舌的两侧出现紫色斑点或舌边青紫；脾胃运化失常，湿浊、

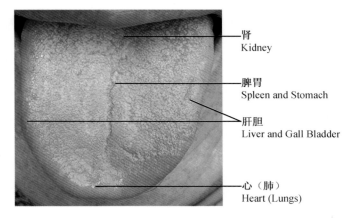

图 1-5

肾
Kidney

脾胃
Spleen and Stomach

肝胆
Liver and Gall Bladder

心（肺）
Heart (Lungs)

痰饮、食滞停积中焦，多见舌中厚腻苔；久病及肾，肾精不足，可见舌根苔剥等等。提示某些脏腑病变在舌象变化上有一定的规律，但并非绝对，还需结合其他症状，加以分析辨别。

二、舌与气血津液的关系

舌为血脉丰富的肌性组织，有赖气血的濡养和津液的滋润。舌体的形质和舌色与气血的盈亏和运行状态有关；舌苔和舌体的润燥与津液的多少有关。

Kidneys store the Essence, Foot Shao Yin Kidney Meridian flows to the root of the tongue; Liver stores Blood, controls the sinews, its channel has a collateral connection with the root of the tongue; the Lung system reaches the throat, having a connection with the root of the tongue. The remaining ZangFu (Zang being the Yin organs and Fu being the Yang organs) are all in some way connected to the tongue either directly or indirectly via connections with the meridians. For this reason, the tongue is a "mirror" that reflects on the condition of the physiological functions. Once pathological changes occur, changes in the tongue will also occur. Therefore, inspecting the various changes of the tongue can predict pathological changes of the internal organs.

The reflection of the internal organs' pathological changes that appear on the surface of the tongue, has a regular pattern of partition. According to the documented history of TCM, amongst them is a more consistent description: the tongue proper signifies the pathological changes of the five Zang, placing emphasis on the Blood system; the tongue coating signifies pathological changes of the six Fu, placing emphasis on the Qi system. The tip of the tongue mainly reflects on pathological changes of the Heart and Lungs of the upper energizer; the center of the tongue mainly reflects on pathological changes of the Stomach and Spleen of the middle energizer; the root of the tongue primarily reflects on pathological changes that occur in the Kidneys of the lower energizer; the borders of the tongue mainly reflect on pathological changes of the Liver and Gall Bladder (Diagram 1-5).

In addition, the text *Grasping Cold-induced Diseases • Inspecting the Tongue and Syndrome Differentiation Method* has another view, stating: "The tip of the tongue belongs to the upper epigastric, the middle of the tongue to the middle epigastric, the root of the tongue to the lower epigastric." In accordance with clinical observations, when there is a flaring-up of heart fire, commonly the tip of the tongue is red or broken (split); in Liver and Gall Bladder Qi stagnation and blood stasis it is common to see purple spots on the borders of the tongue or cyanosis of the borders; a dysfunction of the Spleen and Stomach's role of transformation and transportation, phlegm turbidity, phlegm-fluid retention, food stagnation in the middle energizer, often there is a thick and greasy tongue coating on the center of the tongue; a chronic disease attaining to the Kidneys, deficiency of Kidney Essence can display a peeled coating on the root of the tongue etc, all pointing out that pathological changes of specific organs have a standard pattern of manifestation on the tongue but this is not absolute, therefore it is also important to combine other signs and symptoms to make a differential analysis.

2. The Relationship between the Tongue and Qi, Blood, and Body Fluids

The tongue is the abundant muscular tissue of the blood vessels, dependent on the nourishment from Qi and Blood, and the replenishment and moistening from the Body Fluids. The shape and color of the tongue body is associated with the abundance and the flow of Qi and Blood; the moisture of the tongue coating and the tongue body is more or less connected to the abundance of Body Fluids.

舌下肉阜部有唾液腺腺体的开口，中医认为唾为肾液、涎为脾液，为津液的一部分，其生成、输布离不开脏腑功能，尤其与肾、脾、胃等脏腑密切相关。所以通过观察舌体的润燥，可以判断体内津液的盈亏及病邪性质的寒热。

第三节　舌诊的方法与注意事项

舌诊以望诊为主，还可以结合闻诊、问诊和揩刮等方法进行全面诊察。

一、望舌的体位和伸舌姿势

望舌时患者可采取坐位和仰卧位，但必须使舌面光线明亮，便于观察。伸舌时必须自然地将舌伸出口外，舌体放松，舌面平展，舌尖略向下，尽量张口使舌体充分暴露（图1-6）。

伸舌过分用力，舌体紧张、蜷曲或伸舌时间过长，会影响舌的气血流行而引起舌色、舌苔、干湿度变化（图1-7，1-8，1-9）。

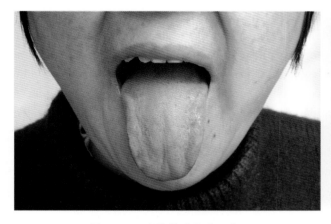

图1-6　正确的伸舌姿式（女）
The correct positioning for extension of the tongue (female)

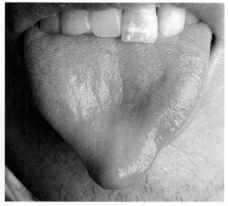

图1-7　不正确的伸舌姿式，舌尖紧缩
（男 室上性心动过速）
Incorrect positioning for extension of the tongue, the tongue tip is tight and shrunken (male, supraventricular tachycardia)

At the underside of the tongue where the sublingual papillae are located are the openings to salivary glands or more specifically the sublingual glands. In TCM, saliva is categorized into two main groups, the slobber (thin saliva) and spittle (thick saliva). Spittle, the fluid of the Kidneys, and slobber the fluid of the Spleen are all a part of the general Body Fluids whose production and distribution rely on the functions of the organs, especially the Kidneys, Spleen, Stomach etc. Therefore through the inspection of the tongue body's moistness or dryness, one can determine abundance or depletion of the Body Fluids and the hot or cold nature of the pathogen.

SECTION THREE   METHODS OF TONGUE DIAGNOSIS AND POINTS OF ATTENTION

Of the Four Examination Methods in TCM, tongue diagnosis belongs to that of looking, that is it is primarily done by observation. When used in combination with the other methods such as, smelling, asking and feeling, it can provide a more complete diagnosis.

1. Positioning of the Body and Extension of the Tongue on Examination

The patient whose tongue is to be examined can either choose to be sitting down or lying down facing upwards, but it is necessary that the tongue is illuminated by light, making it convenient for inspection.

On extension of the tongue it should be done so naturally without excessive force, the tongue should be relaxed in a flat position with the tip of the tongue pointing downwards, and the mouth opens as wide as possible so that the tongue is exposed as much as possible (Diagram 1-6).

If excessive force is used to extend the tongue, the tongue is not relaxed, but curled and if extension time is prolonged, it will affect the flow of Qi and Blood to the tongue, leading to changes of the color, coating and moisture of the tongue (Diagram 1-7, 1-8, 1-9).

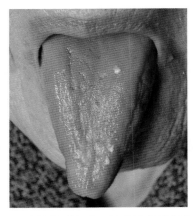

图 1-8　不正确的伸舌姿式，伸舌过度用力致舌色改变
（女　胆囊炎伴结石）
Incorrect positioning for extension of the tongue, excessive force used to extend the tongue causes a change in the tongue color (female, cholecystitis with gallstones)

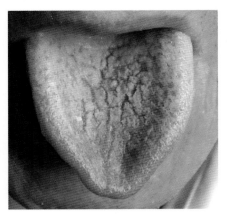

图 1-9　不正确的伸舌姿式，舌边卷屈
（男　消化性溃疡、高血压病）
Incorrect positioning for extension of the tongue, with the tongue borders curled (male, peptic ulcer, hypertension)

二、望舌的方法

望舌的顺序是先看舌尖，再看舌中、舌侧，最后看舌根部；先看舌体的色质，再看舌苔。因为舌质的颜色易变，若伸舌时间过久，舌体易随血管变形而发生色泽变化，导致舌质色泽失真，而舌苔覆盖于舌体上，一般不会随观察的久暂而变化，所以望舌应该先看舌质，再看舌苔。在望舌过程中，既要迅速敏捷，又要全面准确，尽量减少病人的伸舌时间。如果一次望舌判断不清，可令病人休息3～5分钟后，重复望舌一次。

除了通过望诊了解舌象的特征之外，必要时还应配合其他诊察方法。如清·梁玉瑜在《舌鉴辨正》里提出用刮舌验苔的方法进行舌诊，认为刮去浮苔，观察苔底是辨舌的一个重要方面。若刮之不脱或刮而留污质，多为里有实邪；刮之易去，舌体明净光滑则多属虚证。刮舌可用消毒压舌板的边缘，以适中的力量，在舌面上由后向前刮三、五次；如需揩舌，则用消毒纱布裹于手指上，蘸少许生理盐水在舌面上揩抹数次。这两种方法可用于鉴别舌苔有根无根，以及是否属于染苔。

此外，还可询问舌上味觉的情况，舌体有无麻木、疼痛、灼辣等异样感觉。

三、舌诊的注意事项

舌诊是临床诊断疾病的一项重要依据，为了使舌诊所获得的信息准确可靠，就必须讲究望舌的方式方法，注意排除各种操作因素所造成的虚假舌象。

（一）光线的影响

光线的强弱与色调，对颜色的影响极大，稍有疏忽易产生错觉。

2. Method for Inspecting the Tongue

The seguence of inspecting the tongue is first to examine the tip of the tongue, then the middle of the tongue, the borders, and lastly the root of the tongue. The color of the tongue body should first be observed, and then the coating. Because the color of the tongue body alters readily, if there is prolonged extension, the color of the tongue body will change in accordance with the changes to the blood vessels of the tongue, hence the loss of its true color. The tongue coating that covers the tongue body, is not very likely to change due to prolonged extension, thus when inspecting the tongue, the tongue body should first be looked at and then the tongue coating. During the process of examining the tongue, it ought to be done with agility and accuracy, trying best to minimize the time of extension. If assessment of the tongue is not clear on the first attempt, the patient can rest for 3-5 minutes, and thereafter the process repeated.

Apart from observing the tongue to understand the indications of its manifestations, it is also important to combine it with other methods of examination when it is called for. For example, in the Qing Dynasty, Liang Yuyu who compiled *Differentiation of Syndromes by Examination of the Tongue* proposed the method of scraping the tongue and examining the coating, advising that scraping off the superficial tongue coating and inspecting the base coating is one very important aspect. If nothing is removed on scraping or if the coating is still filthy after scraping, this indicates there is most likely an interior excess pathogen; if on scraping, the coating is easily removed and left behind is a clean and smooth tongue body, this usually indicates a deficiency syndrome. The sides of sterile tongue depressors can be used to scrape the tongue, with moderate pressure, on the surface of the tongue from the posterior to the anterior of the tongue three to five times; when it is necessary to scrub the tongue, a sterile cloth wrapped around a finger is dipped in saline solution and used to then scrub the surface of the tongue a few times. These two methods can be used to distinguish whether there is a true or false tongue coating, and also whether the coating is contaminated.

In addition, it is also helpful to inquire about the state of sense of taste, whether there are abnormal sensations such as a feeling of numbness, pain, or hot sensation etc.

3. Points of Attention for Tongue Examination

Tongue examination is an important foundation for diagnosing diseases in clinical practice. For the reliability of accuracy of the information acquired from tongue diagnosis, it is essential to pay much attention to the fashion and method for inspection of the tongue, taking care to eliminate the various operating factors that may lead to false manifestations.

3.1   Effect of Lighting on the Tongue

The strength and color of lighting have an extreme effect on color, where even a slight negligence will result in error.

望舌以白天充足、柔和的自然光线为佳，光线要直接照射到舌面。避免面对有色的光线（图 1-10）。

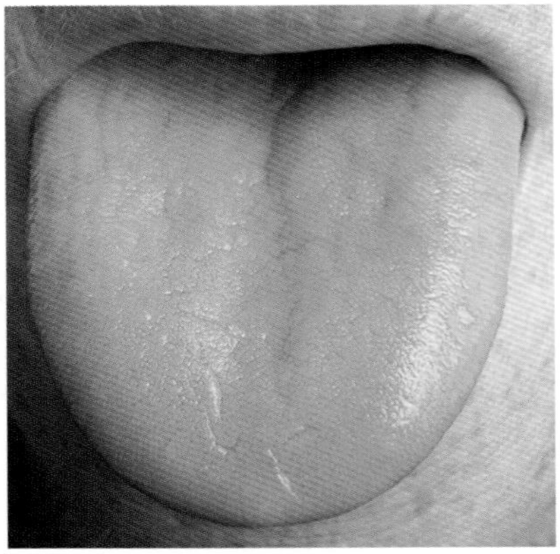

如在夜间或暗处，用日光灯为好。光照的强弱与色调，常常会影响判断的正确性。

如光线过暗，可使舌色暗滞（图 1-11）；用普通的灯泡或手电筒照明，导致舌苔黄白两色难以分辨（图 1-12）；日光灯下，舌色多偏紫；白炽灯下，舌苔偏黄色。周围有色物体的反射光，也会使舌色发生相应的改变（图 1-13，1-14）。

（二）饮食或药品影响

饮食和某些药物可以使舌象发生变化。如进食后，由于口腔咀嚼的摩擦、自洁作用而舌苔由厚变薄；多喝水可使舌苔由燥变润；

图 1-10　自然光线
Under natural sunlight

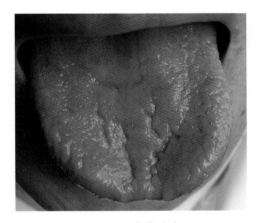

图 1-11　光线过暗
Dull lighting

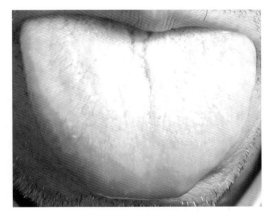

图 1-12　灯光对苔色的影响
Artificial light affecting the coating
making it appear white

过冷过热或刺激性的食物可使舌色发生变化，如刚进辛热食物，舌色偏红（图 1-15）；多吃糖果、甜腻食品、服用大量镇静剂后，可使舌苔厚腻（图 1-16）；长期服用某些抗生素，可产生黑腻苔或霉腐苔（图 1-17）。

某些食物或药物，可以使舌苔着色，称为染苔。

食花生、瓜子、杏仁等富含脂肪的食品，舌面留有黄白色渣滓看似腐腻苔（图 1-18）。

For inspection of the tongue, sunlight that is soft and natural and can directly illuminate the tongue surface is preferred, while colored lights should be avoided (Diagram 1-10).

If inspection is to be done at night or in a dark place, fluorescent light is the best option. The strength of illumination and the color generally affects the accuracy of judgment.

If illumination is too dull, it can make the tongue appear dark in color (Diagram 1-11); the use of a normal light bulb or torch makes it difficult to distinguish between a yellow or white tongue coating (Diagram 1-12); under fluorescent lighting the tongue can appear to be purplish; under incandescent lighting the tongue has a tendency to be yellow in color. Surrounding colored objects that are reflective can also change the tongue color (Diagram 1-13, 1-14).

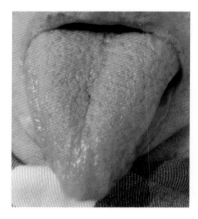

图 1-13　周围有色物体对舌色的影响，舌色偏绿
Surrounding colored objects affecting the color
of the tongue, tongue color appears green.

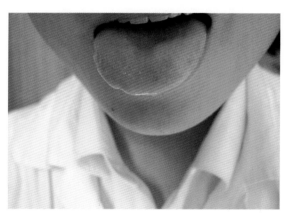

图 1-14　周围有色物体对舌色的影响，舌色偏红
Surrounding colored objects affecting the color
of the tongue, tongue color appears red.

3.2　Effect of Foods or Medicines on the Tongue

Foods and some medications can cause changes to occur in the manifestations of the tongue. For example, after eating, the friction caused by chewing in the oral cavity has a self clean-up action that can cause a thick coating to become thin; imbibing copious amounts of water can cause a dry coating to become moist; excessive consumption of hot, cold, or stimulating foods can cause a change in tongue color; immediately after eating acrid and hot foods, the tongue will appear red (Diagram 1-15); overeating candies, sweets and greasy foods, or taking heavy sedatives can cause the tongue coating to become thick and greasy (Diagram 1-16); long term use of various antibiotics can produce a black and greasy tongue coating or a moldy curd-like coating (Diagram 1-17).

An assortment of foods and medicines can cause a change in color of the tongue coating, which is labeled a contaminated coating.

Consumption of foods containing a high content of fat such as peanuts, melon seeds and almonds etc, leaves yellowish-white remnants or juices on the tongue surface similar to a curd-like and greasy coating(Diagram 1-18).

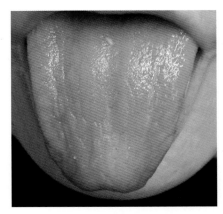

图 1-15　饮食过热使舌色红
Excessive consumption of hot food and
drinks causing the tongue to be red in color.

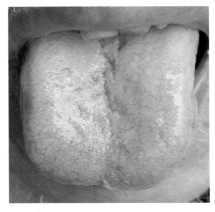

图 1-16　过食甜腻食品舌，苔变厚腻
With excessive consumption of sweet and greasy
foods the tongue coating becomes thick and greasy

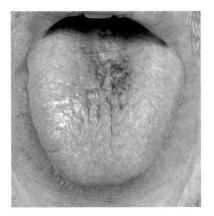

图 1-17　长期服用抗生素，苔色黑黄而腻
After long-term consumption of antibiotics,
coating becomes yellowish black and greasy

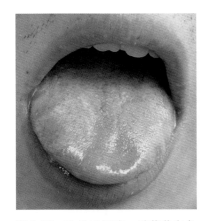

图 1-18　吃瓜子影响，舌苔黄白色
渣滓看似腐腻苔
（Effect of eating melon seeds) Tongue coating is
yellowish white in color and the remnants and juice
remaining appears like a curdy and greasy coating.

　　饮用牛乳、豆浆，舌苔变白、变厚（图 1-19）；蛋黄、橘子，舌苔染成黄色（图
1-20）；各种黑褐色食品、药品，或吃橄榄、酸梅，长期吸烟，使舌苔染成灰色、黑
色（图 1-21）。

（三）口腔对舌象的影响

　　牙齿残缺，可造成同侧舌苔偏厚；镶牙可以使舌边留下齿印；张口呼吸可以使
舌苔变干等等。这些因素引起的舌象异常，都不能作为机体的病理征象，应加以仔
细鉴别，避免误诊。

After drinking cow's milk, soybean milk, the tongue coating becomes white and thick (Diagram 1-19). Eggyolks, oranges make the tongue coating appear yellow (Diagram 1-20). Foods and medicines black in color, olives, plums, and chain smoking, changes the coating to a gray or black color (Diagram 1-21).

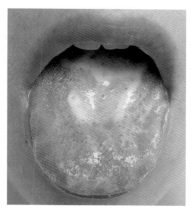

图 1-19　牛奶使苔成白色
Cow milk causes the coating to become white in color.

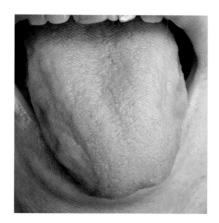

图 1-20　服黄色药物后染成黄色
After the in-take of yellow colored medicine
the coating is contaminated to a yellow color.

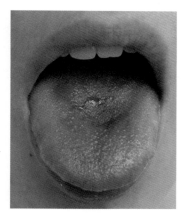

图 1-21　吃巧克力使苔色成褐色
Eating chocolate causes the coating
to become brown in color.

3.3　Effect of the Oral Cavity on the Tongue

A thick coating may appear where there is a fragmented tooth; dentures can leave teeth marks around the edges of the tongue; breathing with the mouth open can cause the coating to become dry etc. These factors that can lead to abnormal changes in the manifestations on a tongue cannot be considered as pathological signs, however, they should be carefully differentiated to avoid error in diagnosis.

第四节　舌诊的内容和正常舌象

一、舌诊的内容

　　舌诊主要观察舌质和舌苔两个方面的变化。舌质是指舌的肌肉脉络组织，为脏腑气血之所荣。望舌质包括舌的颜色、形质和动态及舌下络脉，以候脏腑虚实、气血盛衰与运行情况。舌苔是指舌面上附着的一层苔状物，是胃气上蒸所生。望舌苔包括诊察苔质和苔色情况，以分析病邪的深浅、邪正的消长。《伤寒论本旨·辨舌苔》说："观舌本，可验其正之阴阳虚实。审苔垢，即知邪之寒热浅深。"望诊时，必须综合分析舌质和舌苔，才能对病情有全面了解。

二、正常舌象

　　正常舌象的特征是：舌色淡红鲜明，舌质滋润，舌体柔软灵活；舌苔均匀薄白而润。简称"淡红舌，薄白苔"（图 1-22）。

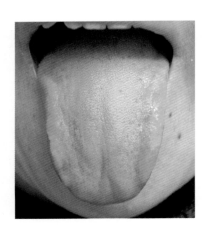

图 1-22　正常舌象
A normal tongue

　　正常舌象的形成原理，文献记载的论述颇多，如《舌鉴总论·白舌总论》说："舌乃心苗，心属火，其色赤，心居肺内，肺属金，其色白，故当舌地淡红，舌苔微白。"《伤寒论本旨·辨舌苔》说："舌苔由胃中生气所现，而胃气由心脾发生。故无病之人常有薄苔，是胃中之生气，如地上之微草也。"《辨舌指南·辨舌质生苔之原理》说："舌之苔，胃蒸脾湿上潮而生。"说明舌象的形成与心、肺、脾、胃等脏腑功能有关。正常舌象提示脏腑机能正常、气血津液充盈、胃气旺盛。

SECTION FOUR   THE CONTENT OF TONGUE DIAGNOSIS AND THE NORMAL TONGUE

1. The Content of Tongue Diagnosis

Tongue diagnosis is carried out by observing changes to the tongue proper and tongue coating. The tongue proper is mainly composed of the tongue muscle and vessels, and is prospered by the Qi and Blood of the Organs. Aspects for inspection of the tongue proper include color, shape, spirit, and the collaterals on the under-side of the tongue to determine the excess or deficiency of the Organs, the prosperity and flow of Qi and Blood. Tongue coating is the moss-like covering that resides over the tongue body; it is the by-product of Stomach Qi steaming up. Aspects for inspection of the tongue coating include the conditions of the tongue coating proper and its color, in order to analyze the depth of a pathogen, and the prosperity or decline of the pathogen and anti-pathogenic Qi. ··· *Interpretation of the Discussion of Cold-Induced Disorders • Differentiating Tongue Coating* states: "Observing the tongue allows the examination of the true state of excess or deficiency of Yin and Yang. Inspecting the coating can determine the hot or cold nature and the depth of the pathogenic factor." When using the looking examination method, it is essential to make a comprehensive analysis of the tongue proper and tongue coating, allowing for a complete understanding of the state of the disease.

2. The Normal Tongue

The characteristics of the normal tongue are: the color of the tongue body should be light red but bright, the tongue proper should appear moist and well nourished, the tongue body should be supple and nimble. The tongue coating should be evenly distributed, thin, white and moist. In a word, it should be "light red tongue, thin white coating" (Diagram 1-22).

There have been considerable discussions from documented literature on the principles for the formation of a normal tongue. As the *General Discussion on Tongue Examination • General Discussion on White Tongues* states: "The tongue is the Sprout of the Heart; Heart pertains to fire, its color is red; the Heart resides within the Lungs, Lung pertains to metal, its color is white, thus the tongue ought to be light red, tongue coating slightly white." *Interpretation of the Discussion of Cold-induced Disorders • Differentiating Tongue Coating* States: "Tongue coating is the manifestation of Qi production in the Stomach, and Stomach Qi is produced with the aid of the Heart and Spleen. Therefore a person without disease mainly has a thin coating, this is the Stomach Producing Qi, like grass growing out of soil." *A Guide to Tongue Differentiation • Principles of Differentiating Tongue Propers and Coating* States: "The coating of the tongue is a result of the Stomach steaming Spleen Dampness upwards." This signifies that the formation of the manifestations of the tongue is related to the physiological functions of the Heart, Lungs, Spleen, Stomach etc. A normal tongue relies on the normal physiological functions of the internal organs, the abundance of Qi, Blood, and Body Fluids, and the prosperity of Stomach Qi.

三、舌象的生理变异

正常的舌象受内外环境影响，可以产生生理性变异。因此，在掌握正常舌象基本特征的前提下，了解生理性变异的特征和原因，及其在健康人群中的分布情况，就可以知常识变，有助于准确判断舌象。

（一）年龄因素

年龄是舌象生理变异的重要因素之一。如儿童阴阳稚弱，脾胃功能尚薄，生长发育很快，往往处于代谢旺盛而营养相对不足的状态，所以舌质多淡嫩，舌苔偏少易剥（图1-23）。老年人精气渐衰，脏腑功能减退，气血运行迟缓，舌色较暗红或带紫暗色（图1-24），但均无明显的病变，故属生理性变异。

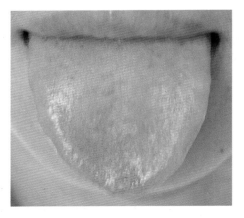

图1-23　舌色淡红，舌质嫩，舌苔薄白
（女　15岁）

Tongue color is light red, tongue proper is
tender, and tongue coating is thin and white
（female，15 years old）

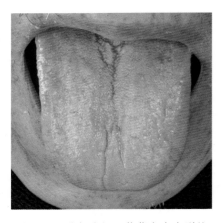

图1-24　舌色暗红，苔薄白中有裂纹
（男　68岁）

Tongue color is dull red, coating is thin
and white with fissures down the middle
（male，68 years old）

（二）性别因素

临床调查资料表明，舌象一般与男女性别无明显关系。但是女性因生理特点，在月经期可以出现蕈状乳头充血而舌质偏红，或舌尖边部点刺增大，月经过后可以恢复正常（图1-25）。

（三）体质、禀赋因素

由于先天禀赋的不同，每个人的体质也不尽相同，舌象可以因此而有差异。《辨舌指南·辨舌之苔垢》说："无病之舌，形色各有不同，有常清洁者，有稍生苔层者，有鲜红者，有淡白色者，或为紧而尖，或为松而软，并有牙印者……此因无病时各有禀体之不同，故舌质亦异也。"提示因禀赋体质不同，可以出现一些异常舌

3. The Physiological Changes of the Tongue

The normal tongue can be influenced by its internal or external environment, which would lead to changes of its physiological nature. Therefore, based on understanding the normal tongue and its basic characteristics, it is important to discern the principles and characteristics of its physiological changes, and the situation of its distribution amongst the healthy in order to identify the norm and recognize changes subsequently contributing to a more precise judgment of the tongue.

3.1   Age Factor

Age is one of the important factors that influence physiological changes of the tongue. For example, in infants Yin and Yang are immature with the functions of the Spleen and Stomach still weak. Meanwhile growth and development is rapid, metabolism is thriving while nourishment is inadequate. Therefore children's tongues are paler and more tender, the tongue coating tends to be less and prone to peeling (Diagram 1-23). Amongst the elderly the Qi and Essence are progressively deteriorating with the functions of the organs declining, the flow and transportation of Qi and Blood sluggish and tongue color relatively dull or dull purplish (Diagram 1-24). However, for the above mentioned there is no apparent pathological change, therefore they are considered physiological changes.

3.2   Sex Factor

Data obtained from clinical observations have indicated that there is no significant relation between sex and manifestations of the tongue, but for females due to distinctive physiological aspects during menstruation flow, the fungiform papillae become filled with blood. Therefore the tongue proper has a tendency to be red, or the speckles on the tip and borders of the tongue become enlarged. As the menstruation pass, the tongue can return to normal (Diagram 1-25).

3.3   Constitution and Innate Factor

Due to the difference in the pre-heavenly innateness, every individual's constitution will also differ to an extent. For this reason, there will be discrepancies in the manifestations of the tongue. *A Guide to Tongue Differentiation • Differentiating Turbid Coatings of the Tongue* states: "Non-diseased tongues can differ in form and color. There are clean tongues, those with slight production of coating, those that are bright red, those that are a pale white color, or stiff and pointy, or loose and soft, and also those with teeth marks, ···this is due to the difference in the innate constitution when there is an absence of disease, thus the tongue proper is also different." This signifies that the variation in the innate constitution can emerge in atypical manifestations of the tongue. In clinical practice it is common to see enlarged, plump and pale tongues in people who are overweight (Diagram 1-26), whereas thin,

象。临床常见肥胖之人舌多胖大而质淡（图1-26），消瘦之人舌体偏瘦而舌色偏红（图1-27）。

除上述外，尚有先天性裂纹舌、齿痕舌、地图舌等（图1-28，1-29，1-30），多见于禀赋不足、体质较弱者。虽长期无明显临床症状，但可以表现出对某些病邪的易感性，或某些疾病的好发性。

（四）气候因素

气候随着季节与地域的差别而变化，

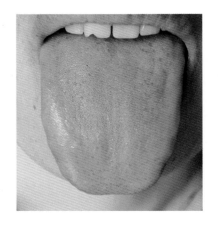

图1-25 月经期 舌色红，
舌面有芒刺，苔薄（女）
During menstruation the tongue is red in color
with prickles on the surface of the tongue,
and a thin coating (female)

舌象相应发生改变，反映了人的生理活动与自然界息息相关的天人相应的思想。

季节方面：夏季暑湿盛行，舌苔多厚，色偏黄（图1-31）；秋季燥气当令，舌多偏干（图1-32）；冬季严寒，舌多湿润（图1-33）。地域方面：我国东南地区偏热偏湿，西北及东北地区偏寒偏燥，舌象会相应发生一定的变异（图1-34）。

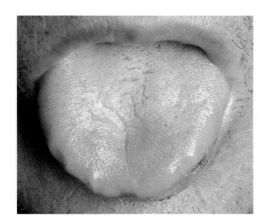

图1-26 胖人之舌 舌色紫，舌边有齿痕，
苔淡黄腻（男）
The tongue of an overweight person is
purplish in color, with tooth-marked borders,
and a pale yellow and greasy coating (male)

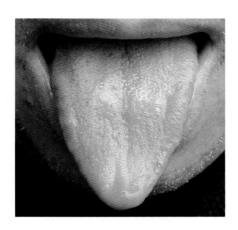

图1-27 瘦人之舌 舌色红，
舌体瘦薄，苔薄黄（男）
The tongue of an underweight person is red in
color, the tongue body is thin and emaciated
with and a thin yellow coating (male)

red tongues are frequently seen in people who are underweight (Diagram 1-27).

Apart from the above mentioned, there are also inherent cracked tongues, tooth-marked tongues, and mapped tongues etc (Diagram 1-28, 1-29, 1-30). which mostly occur when the innate factor is deficient, and the constitution is comparatively weak. Although there may not be any apparent clinical signs or symptoms, it can present itself by being susceptible to certain pathogens, or to the occurrence of particular diseases.

3.4   Climatic Factor

The changes in the climate are in accordance with the variation in seasonal and geographical aspects, which also corresponds to the changes in the manifestations of the tongue, reflecting the "Union of Heaven and Man" thought that there is an intimate relationship between the physiological activity and life of human beings and their natural environment.

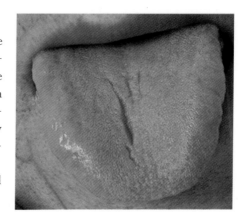

图 1-28　舌色暗红，舌中有裂纹，
苔薄（男）
A dull red tongue with cracks down
the midline, and a thin coating (male)

Seasonal aspect: In summer, summer-heat and dampness are thriving, tongue coating is thicker, and the color tends to be yellow (Diagram 1-31). Autumn is the season for dryness, so the tongue has a tendency to be dry (Diagram 1-32). In winter it is rigorously cold, so the tongue is more damp and moist (Diagram 1-33). Geographical aspect: In China, in the South Eastern regions, it tends to be damp and hot, while the North Western and North Eastern regions tend to be cold and dry, hence specified changes in the tongue will occur correspondingly (Diagram 1-34).

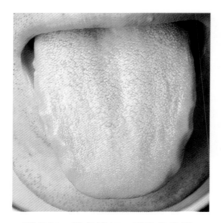

图 1-29　舌色淡红，舌边有齿痕，
苔淡黄（男）
A light red tongue, with tooth-marked tongue
borders and a pale yellow coating (male)

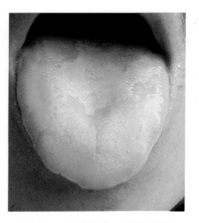

图 1-30　舌质淡嫩，舌苔剥落，
边界清楚（男）
A pale and tender tongue and peeled tongue
coating, with the edges clearly visible (male)

　　此外，因为舌象能灵敏地反映机体内部的病变，舌象变化可早于自觉症状而出现，因此，若正常人出现异常舌象，除了上述生理因素外，有一部分可能是疾病前期的征象。所以应把真正的生理变异与病变前期的病态舌象区分开来。一般说来，异常舌象长期不变，无任何不适症状出现，属于生理性变异；否则应考虑是疾病的前期病变，可以通过问诊加以区别，必要时进行随访后再作出判断。

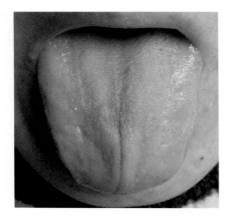

图 1-31　夏季舌苔偏黄
（男）

In the summer the tongue coating
has a tendency to be yellow（male）

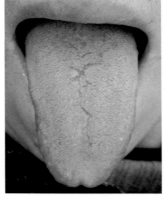

图 1-32　秋季舌苔偏干，舌色红，
舌苔黄而燥（女）

In autumn, the tongue coating tends to be dry
and yellow, and the tongue red in color（female）

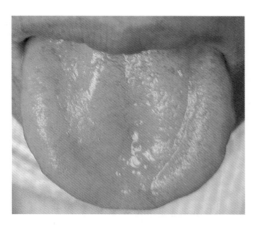

图 1-33　舌色淡红，舌面润泽，冬季舌苔湿润
（女）

A light red tongue, and a tongue surface
that is moist. In winter the tongue
coating is damp（female）

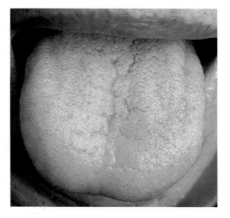

图 1-34　地域对舌象的影响，东南地区苔多黄腻，
舌色红，舌苔黄腻（男）

Geographical aspects affect the tongue.
In the South Eastern regions, the coating is
mostly yellow and greasy, tongue is red,
and tongue coating is yellow and greasy（male）

Moreover, because the tongue manifestations can insightfully reflect on pathological changes in the body, changes in the tongue can appear earlier than when the patient experiences other symptoms. Therefore, if there are changes in the manifestations of a tongue in a normal person, except for the above physiological factors, it can be a forewarning sign to disease for some individuals. For this reason, it is vital to differentiate whether the manifestations of the tongue are due to changes in the physiological factors or a premonitory sign of disease. Generally speaking, the continual presence of an abnormal presentation of the tongue, unless accompanied by any other abnormal signs or symptoms, can be diagnosed as physiological changes. If this is not the case, then it should be considered that a premonitory sign of a disease is possible. In this case, the use of other diagnostic methods such as interrogation can be utilized in conjunction to differentiate. When necessary, a judgment can be made after the examination.

第二章

望 舌 质

　　舌质，即舌的本体，故又称舌体，是舌的肌肉和脉络组织。望舌体主要观察舌神、舌色、舌的形质、动态以及舌下络脉5个部分。

第一节　舌　神

　　舌神，即舌的荣枯、润燥及舌的色泽，一般分为荣舌、枯舌两种。

一、荣舌

　　【舌象特征】　舌质荣润红活，鲜明，有生气、有光彩为荣舌（图2-1）。
　　【临床意义】　是机体正气充盛的标志之一。
　　【机理分析】　《辨舌指南·辨舌之神气》说："荣润则津足，干枯则津乏。荣者谓有神……凡舌质有光有体，不论黄、白、灰、黑，刮之而里面红润，神气荣华者，诸病皆吉。"

二、枯舌

　　【舌象特征】　舌质干枯死板，色泽晦暗，没有光泽，为枯舌（图2-2）。
　　【临床意义】　疾病严重、预后不良的标志之一。

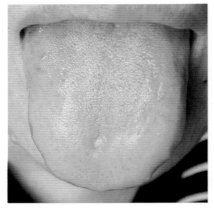

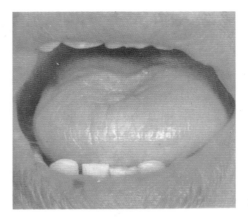

图2-1　荣舌舌色淡红，苔薄
（女　正常人）
A flourishing tongue which is light red in color,
and has a thin coating (female, healthy individual)

图2-2　舌色枯白，毫无光泽
（男　胃癌）
Tongue is ashen in color with no vitality
(male, stomach cancer)

CHAPTER TWO

INSPECTING THE TONGUE PROPER

The tongue proper, also called the tongue body, is constructed of muscles and collaterals. Inspection of the tongue mainly involves observing 5 aspects pertaining to itself: the vitality, the color, the body shape, the movements of the tongue, and the vessels on the underside of the tongue.

SECTION ONE   TONGUE SPIRIT

Tongue spirit, which is also the vitality of the tongue, includes its moisture and the color of the tongue, It is primarily separated into two types: flourishing tongue and withered tongue.

1. Flourishing Tongue

Characteristics: A flourishing tongue is where the tongue proper is flourishing, moist, bright, fresh and red, has "life", and vitality (Diagram 2-1).

Clinical Significance: It is an indication of the state of the anti-pathogenic Qi.

Pathogenesis Analysis: *A Guide to Tongue Differentiation · Differentiating the Spirit of the Tongue* states: "A flourishing and moist tongue indicates sufficiency of body fluids, while a dry and ashen tongue indicates the exhaustion of body fluids. Flourishing means having 'spirit', the tongue proper having vitality and substance. If the spirit is flourishing and prosperous, whether its color is yellow, white, gray, or black, on scraping the tongue the interior is red and moist, the fate of the disease is good. "

2. Ashen Tongue

Characteristics: An ashen tongue is where the tongue proper is dry, ashen and lacking vitality and brightness, has no "life"; the color is dark and dull (Diagram 2-2).

Clinical Significance: It is an indication of severe diseases, and poor prognosis.

【机理分析】《辨舌指南·辨舌之神气》说："荣润则津足，干枯则津乏……若舌质无光无体，不拘有苔无苔，视之里面枯晦，神气全无者，诸病皆凶。"

第二节 舌 色

舌色，即舌体的颜色。一般分为淡红、淡白、红、红绛、青紫5种。

一、淡红舌

【舌象特征】 舌体颜色淡红润泽，白中透红（图2-3）。

【临床意义】 淡红舌为气血调和的征象，常见于正常人。病中见之多属病轻。

【机理分析】 淡红舌主要反映心之气血充足、胃气旺盛的生理状态。舌色与肤色的形成原理相似，红为血之色，明润光泽为胃气之华，正如《舌苔统志·淡红舌》所说："舌色淡红，平人之常候，……红者心之气，淡者胃之气。"

外感病初起，病情轻浅，尚未伤及气血及内脏时，舌色仍可保持正常而呈淡红；内伤疾病时见之，提示阴阳平和，气血充盈，多属病轻，或为疾病转愈之象。

二、淡白舌

【舌象特征】 舌色比正常浅淡，白色偏多，红色偏少（图2-4）。

【临床意义】 多主气血两虚、阳虚。

【机理分析】 因气血亏虚，血不荣舌，或阳气虚衰，运血无力，无以推动血液上充于舌，致舌色浅淡。

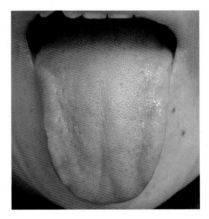

图 2-3 舌色淡红，苔薄白
（女 正常人）

Tongue is light red in color, and coating is
thin and white (female, healthy individual)

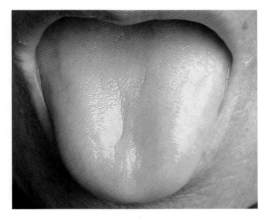

图 2-4 舌色淡白，舌苔根部淡黄腻
（女 急性粒细胞白血病）

Tongue is palewhite in color, and tongue
coating at the root is pale yellow and greasy
(female, acute granulocytic leukemia)

Pathogenesis Analysis: *A Guide to Tongue Differentation • Differentiating the Spirit of the Tongue* states. "Flourishing and moist indicates the abundance of body fluids, while dry and ashen indicates depletion of body fluids ⋯ If a tongue is ashen, dark and totally lacking of spirit, vitality or substance, there is an indication of ill fate of the disease, whether the coating is present or not."

SECTION TWO   TONGUE COLOR

The tongue color refers to the color of the tongue body. Generally there are five colors: light red, pale, red, dark red, blue and purple.

1. Light Red Tongue

Characteristics: The color of the tongue body is light red, lustrous and moist, white with red seeping through (Diagram 2-3).

Clinical Significance: A light red tongue is a sign of harmony of Qi and Blood, generally seen in normal healthy individuals. If seen during a disease, it indicates that the disease is mild.

Pathogenesis Analysis: The light red tongue mainly reflects the physiology where the Heart Qi and Blood are sufficient and Stomach Qi is thriving. The principle for the formation of tongue color is similar to that of skin color, where red is the color of blood, and the flourishing of Stomach Qi gives it its luster and vitality. According to *A Collection of Tongues and Coatings • Light Red Tongue* "A light red tongue is the manifestation of the common people, ⋯red being Qi of the Heart, and light red being Qi of the Stomach."

During the early stages of an externally-contracted disease where the syndrome is mild and in the superficial level, and where there has been no injury done to the Qi, Blood, or internal organs, the color of the tongue can still remain as normal, appearing as light red in color; when seen in an internal impairment disease, it denotes the harmony of Yin and Yang, the exuberance of Qi and Blood, mostly indicating a mild syndrome, or a sign that a disease has undergone a change for the better to recovery.

2. Pale Tongue

Characteristics: The color is paler than that of a normal tongue with the white color more obvious than the red color (Diagram 2-4).

Clinical Significance: Indicative of Qi and Blood deficiency, or Yang Qi deficiency.

Pathogenesis Analysis: Due to the deficiency of Qi and Blood, the Blood does not flourish the tongue, or the deficiency of Yang Qi does not have the ability to transport the Blood, cannot move the Blood to reach the tongue, therefore causing a pale tongue.

淡白舌根据舌色的荣、枯及舌的形状一般分为淡白胖舌、淡白瘦舌、枯白舌3种。

（一）淡白胖舌

【舌象特征】 舌色淡白而舌体胖嫩（图 2-5）。

【临床意义】 主阳气虚。

【机理分析】 阳虚则内寒，经脉收引，使舌的血行减少，也可见舌淡。《舌鉴辨正·白舌总论》指出，淡白舌是"虚寒舌之本色"。若淡白湿润，舌体胖嫩，多属阳虚水停。

（二）淡白瘦舌

【舌象特征】 舌色淡白而舌体瘦薄（图 2-6）。

【临床意义】 主气血不足。

【机理分析】 舌色淡而舌体瘦薄，属气血两虚，血不上荣所致。

（三）枯白舌

【舌象特征】 舌体色白，全无血色，则称为枯白舌（图 2-7）。

【临床意义】 枯白舌主伤精、脱血夺气。

【机理分析】 提示病情危重。精血耗竭、脱血夺气，无以荣舌，故见舌枯白无华。

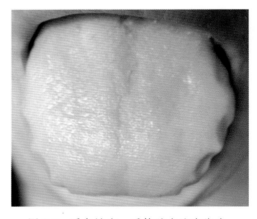

图 2-5 舌色淡白，舌体胖大边有齿痕，舌苔薄（男 再生障碍性贫血）
Tongue color is pale white, tongue body is puffy and swollen with teeth-marks, and a thin tongue coating (male, aplastic anemia)

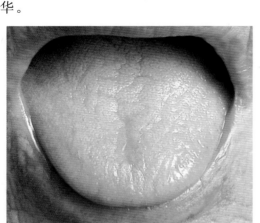

图 2-6 舌色淡，舌体瘦小，舌苔薄白（男 慢性胃炎）
The tongue is pale, the tongue body is emaciated, with a thin and white tongue coating (male, chronic gastritis)

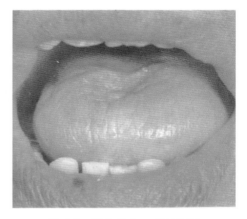

图 2-7 舌色枯白，毫无光泽（男 胃癌）
The tongue is ashen and white with no vitality (male, stomach cancer)

A pale white tongue is further categorized, according to its vitality, moisture and form, generally into 3 types: a pale white and enlarged tongue, pale white and thin tongue, or a withered and white tongue.

2. 1   Pale and Puffy Tongue

Characteristics: The tongue is pale, puffy and tender (Diagram 2-5).

Clinical Significance: Indicative of Yang Qi deficiency.

Pathogenesis Analysis: A deficiency of Yang Qi leads to internal cold, causing contractions in the meridians, and depleting the flow of Blood in the tongue, and can also appear as a pale tongue. *Differentiation of Syndromes by Examination of the tongue • General Discussion on white Tongue* points out that a pale tongue is "the basic color of a deficiency cold tongue". If it is pale and moist, and the body is puffy and tender, it is mainly indicative of Yang deficiency with accumulation of fluids.

2. 2   Pale and Thin Tongue

Characteristics: The tongue is pale and thin (Diagram 2-6).

Clinical Significance: Indicative of the insufficiency of Qi and Blood.

Pathogenesis Analysis: Due to the insufficiency of Qi and Blood, the Blood fails to arise to nourish the tongue.

2. 3   Ashen and White Tongue

Characteristics: The color of the tongue is white, completely devoid of blood color, which is labeled an ashen and white tongue (Diagram 2-7).

Clinical Significance: Indicative of injury to the Essence, the prostration of Blood and collapse of Qi.

Pathogenesis Analysis: Signifies an extremely severe syndrome. The exhaustion of Blood and the Essence, the prostration of Blood and collapse of Qi fails to flourish the tongue, hence the appearance of a dull and white tongue without luster.

三、红舌

【舌象特征】　舌色较正常舌色红，呈鲜红者，称为红舌（图2-8，2-9）。

【临床意义】　主实热、阴虚内热。

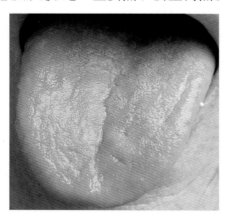

图 2-8　舌色红，前部少苔根部淡腻
（男　十二指肠溃疡）
Tongue color is red，the anterior of the tongue has
scanty coating and the coating at the root is pale
and greasy (male, duodenal ulcer)

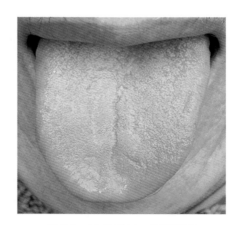

图 2-9　舌色鲜红，舌苔薄黄
（男　肺部感染）
Tongue is bright red in color，with a thin and
yellow tongue coating (male, pneumonia)

【机理分析】　血得热则行，热使血管扩张、血行加速，热使气血沸涌，致使舌体脉络充盈而舌色鲜红；或阴虚水涸，虚火上炎于舌络而舌红。

红舌根据舌色所反映的部位及舌苔的多少、舌形的变化，一般分为舌尖红、舌边红、舌色鲜红兼黄厚苔、舌色鲜红少苔4种。

（一）舌尖红

【舌象特征】　舌尖颜色比舌体偏红（图2-10）。

【临床意义】　提示外感表热证初起或心火上炎。

【机理分析】　舌尖为心肺所主，舌尖红为心火上炎或风热表证。

（二）舌两边红赤

【舌象特征】　舌体两边颜色红赤（图2-11）。

【临床意义】　多为肝胆热盛。

【机理分析】　舌两边为肝胆所主，肝胆热盛，故见舌两边红赤。

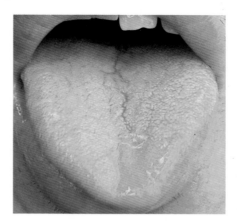

图 2-10　舌尖红，舌苔黄白相间
（男　失眠待查）
A red tongue tip，with a yellow and white tongue
coating (male, insomnia awaiting examination)

3. Red Tongue

Characteristics: This is a color that is redder than the normal tongue, appears as a bright fresh red color, and thus is named a red tongue (Diagram 2-8, 2-9).

Clinical Significance: Indicative of excess heat, or Yin deficiency and internal heat.

Pathogenesis Analysis: When Blood receives heat, it moves. Heat will enlarge the blood vessels, making blood flow become more rapid, and compel Qi and Blood to boil and gush, instigating the superabundance of the collaterals of the tongue so that the tongue color is bright red; or Yin deficiency and drying up of fluids, the flaring up of deficient fire to the collaterals of the tongue causing a red tongue.

A red tongue is primarily categorized according to the partition of the red color on the tongue, the quantity of tongue coating, and changes in the tongue shape. Generally there are four categories, red tongue tip, red tongue borders, bright red tongue with thick yellow coating, bright red tongue with scanty coating.

3.1   Red Tongue Tip

Characteristics: The color of the tongue tip is comparatively redder than the tongue body (Diagram 2-10).

Clinical Significance: Signifying the early stages of a superficial externally contracted heat syndrome or the flaring up of Heart fire.

Pathogenesis Analysis: As the tip of the tongue corresponds to the Heart and Lungs, thus if the tip of the tongue is red, it indicates Heart fire flaring up or exterior wind heat syndrome.

3.2   Red Tongue Borders

Characteristics: The two sides of the tongue body are red in color (Diagram 2-11).

Clinical Significance: Chiefly indicating exuberant heat in the Liver and Gallbladder.

Pathogenesis Analysis: The two sides or borders of the tongue corresponds to the Liver and Gall Bladder, when there is exuberant heat in the Liver and Gall Bladder, hence the redness of the borders of the tongue.

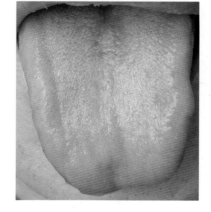

图 2-11   舌两边红赤，苔薄黄
（男   高血压，2 型糖尿病）

Red tongue borders on both sides, with a thin yellow coating (male, hypertension and type II diabetes)

（三）舌色鲜红兼黄厚苔

【舌象特征】 舌体大小不变，舌色鲜红兼黄厚苔（图 2-12）。

【临床意义】 属实热证。

【机理分析】 舌色红而有苔者，多属实热证，多为热使血管扩张，故舌色见红，热虽盛，胃阴未伤，故舌仍有苔。

（四）舌色鲜红少苔

【舌象特征】 舌色鲜红少苔，或伴有裂纹，或光红无苔，舌体瘦小者（图 2-13，2-14，2-15）。

【临床意义】 多为虚热证。

【机理分析】 舌色鲜红少苔或有裂纹、舌体瘦小多为虚热证。《辨舌指南·辨舌之颜色》说："舌色鲜红，无苔点，舌底无津，舌面无液者，阴虚火炎也。"

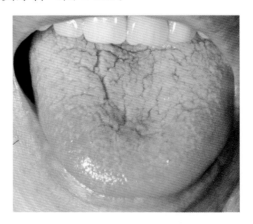

图 2-12 舌色红，舌边肿胀，苔黄腐厚
（男 脑供血不足）
A red tongue, with swollen tongue borders,
and a thick yellow and curdy coating
(male, insufficient blood-supply to the brain)

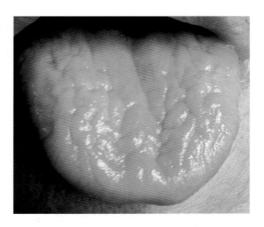

图 2-13 舌色红，舌质嫩，舌面有裂纹
（男 支气管炎）
A red and tender tongue, with fissures on the
the tongue surface (male, bronchitis)

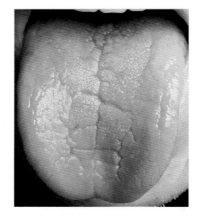

图 2-14 舌色红，舌面裂纹，苔薄白
（男 左下肺感染）
A red tongue, with fissures on the tongue surface,
and a thin white coating (male, pneumonia of the
lower lobe of the left Lung)

四、绛舌

【舌象特征】 舌色较红舌的红色更深，称为绛舌（图 2-16）。

【临床意义】 多主里热亢盛，阴虚火旺。

3.3 Bright Red Tongue with a Thick Yellow Coating

Characteristics: There is no change in the size of the tongue, tongue color is bright red and the tongue coating is thick and yellow (Diagram 2-12).

Clinical Significance: Indicating an excessive heat syndrome.

Pathogenesis Analysis: When the tongue is red and there is presence of a coating, this generally signifies an excessive heat syndrome, chiefly being the enlargement of the blood vessels due to heat, hence the red tongue body. Although there is an exuberance of heat, the Stomach Yin is not yet to be impaired, thus the presence of tongue coating.

3.4 Bright Red Tongue with Scanty Coating

Characteristics: Tongue color is bright red with scanty coating, or accompanied by cracks, or bright red color with no coating, and thin tongue body (Diagram 2-13, 2-14, 2-15).

Clinical Significance: Primarily indicating a deficiency heat syndrome.

Pathogenesis Analysis: This kind of the tongue primarily indicates a deficiency heat syndrome. *A Guide to Tongue Differentiation • Differentiating Colors of the Tongue* states: "Color of the tongue that is bright red, without coating or spots, absence of fluids on the underside and surface of the tongue, indicates Yin deficiency with flaring up of fire."

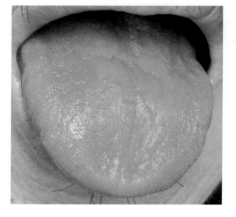

图 2-15 舌鲜红，舌体瘦小薄无苔
（男 胃癌广泛转移）
The tongue is bright red, tongue body is thin
and emaciated with the absence of coating
(male, extensive metastases of stomach cancer)

4. Deep Red Tongue

Characteristics: When the redness is darker than that of a red tongue, it is a deep red tongue (Diagram 2-16).

Clinical Significance: Indicates an exuberance of interior heat or Yin deficiency with exuberant fire.

【机理分析】 绛舌多由红舌进一步发展而成。其形成原因一是邪热亢盛，气血沸涌，舌部血络充盈而舌红绛；二是因热入营血，耗伤营阴，血液浓缩，血热充斥于舌而舌绛；三是可因阴虚水涸，虚火上炎于舌络而舌红。所以，绛舌比红舌的病情深重。

绛舌根据舌色的浅深及舌苔的多少、有无，一般分为舌色红绛而有苔、舌色红绛而少苔或无苔2种。

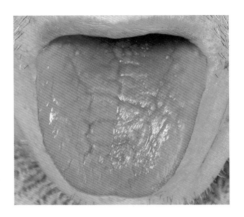

图 2-16 舌红绛，无苔，舌面有纵行裂纹
（男 食管癌）
A deep red tongue, absence of coating, and horizontal fissures on the tongue surface
(male, esophageal cancer)

（一）舌色红绛而有苔

【舌象特征】 舌色红绛而有苔（图 2-17，2-18）。

【临床意义】 主实热证。

【机理分析】 舌色红绛而有苔者，多由外感热病，热入营血，或内伤杂病，脏腑阳热偏盛所致。

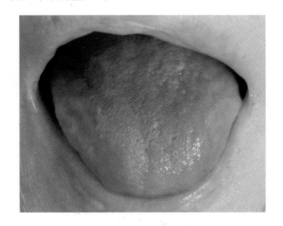

图 2-17 舌色红绛，苔色白
（女 脑梗塞）
A deepred tongue, with a white coating
(female, cerebral infarction)

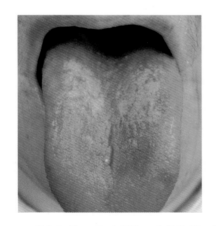

图 2-18 舌色红绛，舌面干燥，舌苔前部、根部少苔，中部有少量淡黄苔（男 高血压病）
A deep red tongue, with a dry tongue surface, scanty coating on the anterior and root of the tongue, and a small amount of pale yellow coating on the centre of the tongue (male, hypertension)

（二）舌色红绛而少苔或无苔

【舌象特征】 舌色红绛而少苔或无苔（图 2-19）。

【临床意义】 提示胃、肾阴伤。

Pathogenesis Analysis: A deep red tongue is typically a further progression of the red tongue. Its conception is firstly due to the exuberance of pathogenic heat, leading to the gushing of Qi and Blood, overflowing to the collaterals of the tongue hence the deep red color of the tongue; secondly it is due to pathogenic heat entering the nutritive and blood levels, injuring the nutritive Yin, concentration of Blood, heat in the blood floods to the tongue causing the deep red tongue; and thirdly Yin deficiency and the drying up of fluids, deficiency fire flaring up to the collaterals of the tongue and causing the deep red color. Thus a deep red tongue in comparison to a red tongue indicates a more severe syndrome.

A deep red tongue is classified by the color intensity of the tongue and the presence or absence of a tongue coating mainly into 2 groups: a deep red tongue with coating, and deep red tongue with scanty coating or no coating.

4.1 Deep Red Tongue with Coating

Characteristics: The tongue is a deep red color and there is a presence of coating (Diagram 2-17, 2-18).

Clinical Significance: Indicates an excessive heat syndrome.

Pathogenesis Analysis: Mainly signifying an externally contracted heat syndrome entering the nutritive and blood levels or a miscellaneous internal impairment syndrome, due to the exuberance of the Yang heat internal organs.

4.2 Deep Red Tongue with Scanty Coating or No Coating

Characteristics: The tongue is a deep red color with scanty coating or without coating (Diagram 2-19).

Clinical Significance: Indicating the impairment of Stomach and Kidney Yin.

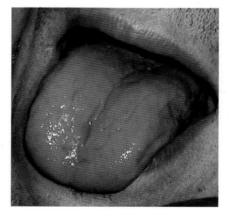

图 2-19 舌色红绛，舌体胖嫩，
舌面无苔（男 高血压病）

A deep red tongue, with a puffy and tender tongue body, and absence of coating (male, hypertension)

【机理分析】《辨舌指南·辨舌之颜色》说："绛，深红色也。心主营、主血。舌苔绛燥，邪已入营中。""绛而光亮者，胃阴亡也。""舌虽绛而不鲜，干枯而痿者，肾阴涸也。"舌色红绛而少苔或无苔者，提示胃、肾阴伤，多由热病后期阴液受损，或久病阴虚火旺所致，属虚热证。

五、青紫舌

【舌象特征】 全舌呈均匀青色或紫色，或局部现青紫色斑点，均称青紫舌（图2-20，2-21）。

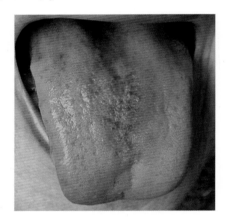

图 2-20 舌色暗紫，苔色黄
（女 冠状动脉粥样硬化性心脏病）
Tongue is dull purple in color, with a yellow coating
(female, coronary atherosclerotic heart disease)

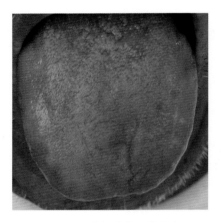

图 2-21 舌色暗紫，苔色白
（男 肾病综合征）
Tongue is dull purple in color, and a white
coating (male, nephrotic syndrome)

【临床意义】 主气血运行不畅。

【机理分析】 舌紫色的深浅与寒热性质有关。紫舌是气血运行不畅所致。全舌青紫，表明瘀血较重，多是全身性瘀血所致；舌有紫色斑点者，瘀血程度较轻，多见于瘀血阻滞局部，或局部脉络损伤所致。青紫舌还可见于某些先天性心脏病，或药物、食物中毒等病证。

青紫舌根据紫色的浅深及舌苔润燥，一般分为淡青紫舌，紫红、绛紫舌，瘀斑舌、瘀点舌 3 类。

（一）淡青紫舌

【舌象特征】 舌淡而泛现青紫色，则为淡青紫舌（图2-22）。

【临床意义】 阴寒内盛或阳气虚衰。

【机理分析】 舌色淡紫或紫暗而湿润，多见于阳虚阴盛之证，多由阴寒内盛，阳气不宣，气血不畅，血脉瘀滞而致；舌色青为寒凝血瘀之重证，提示阴寒内盛，阳气受遏，血行凝滞。

Pathogenesis Analysis: *A Guide to Tongue Differentiation* • *Differentiating colors of the Tongue* states: "Deep red is a dark red color. The Heart governs the nutritive and the Blood. A deep red tongue and dry coating signifies the pathogen has entered the nutritive level." "Deep red color that is bright and shiny indicates the collapse of Stomach Yin", "The tongue is deep red but not bright, is dried, withered and flaccid, indicating the exhaustion of Kidney Yin." A deep red tongue with scanty coating or no coating indicates the impairment of Stomach and Kidney Yin due to the late stages of a febrile disease where the Yin and body fluids are injured, or a chronic disease leading to Yin deficiency and fire flaring up, pertaining to deficiency heat syndrome.

5. Cyanosed Tongue

Characteristics: Cyanosed tongue refers to the entire tongue being evenly distributed with a blue or purple color or a part of the tongue that is bluish-purple in color with purple spots (Diagram 2-20、2-21).

Clinical Significance: Indicative of the obstructive flow of Qi and Blood.

Pathogenesis Analysis: The color intensity of a purple tongue is related to the nature of heat and cold. A purple tongue is the result of an obstructive flow of Qi and Blood. Cyanosis of the entire tongue indicates severe blood stasis, mainly referring to generalized blood stasis of the whole body. A tongue with purple spots indicates the blood stasis is rather mild, mainly referring to localized blood stasis, or injury to a localized area of a meridian. Cyanosis of the tongue can also be seen in some inherited Heart diseases, or poisoning from medications, and foods etc.

A cyanotic tongue is categorized according to the intensity of the purple color as well as the moisture of the tongue coating. It is generally divided into 3 groups, pale cyanotic tongue, purplish red or purplish deep red tongue, tongue with ecchymoses, or tongue with purple spots.

5.1   Pale Cyanosis of the Tongue

Characteristics: The tongue is pale yet suffused with a cyanosis color, thus the label pale cyanosis of the tongue (Diagram 2-22).

Clinical Significance: Indicative of exuberance internal cold or Yang deficiency.

Pathogenesis Analysis: A pale purple or dull purple tongue that is moist is primarily seen in deficiency Yang and excess Yin syndromes. Generally exuberant internal cold, makes Yang Qi unable to disperse, leading to the sluggish flow of Qi and Blood, and blood stasis in the blood vessels; a blue tongue indicates a severe syndrome of blood stasis due to cold congealment and exuberance of internal Yin and cold restraining Yang and coagulating Blood.

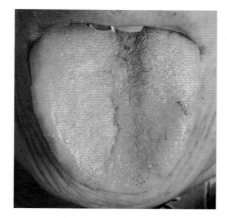

图 2-22   舌淡紫，苔白
（女   贫血待查）

A pale purple tongue, and a white coating
(female, anemia awaiting examination)

（二）紫红、绛紫舌

【舌象特征】　舌红而泛现紫色，则为紫红舌（图 2-23）；舌绛而泛现紫色，则为绛紫舌（图 2-24）。

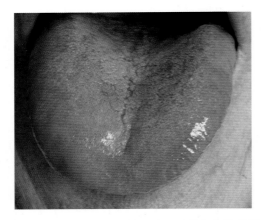

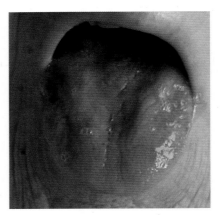

图 2-23　舌色紫红，舌体肿胀，舌苔根部淡黄腻
（男　原发性支气管肺癌）

A purplish red and swollen tongue, and a pale
yellow and greasy tongue coating at the root
(male, primary bronchogenic carcinoma)

图 2-24　舌色绛并泛现紫色，舌面水滑苔
（女　肝硬化）

A deep red tongue appearing purplish red, and a
watery and slippery coating on the tongue surface
(female, hepatocirrhosis)

【临床意义】　热毒炽盛，气血壅滞。

【机理分析】　舌色紫暗或绛紫而干枯少津，舌苔少而干，多见于热证，提示热毒炽盛，深入营血，营阴受灼，气血不畅。

（三）瘀斑舌、瘀点舌

【舌象特征】　舌上局部出现青紫色斑点，大小不一，不高于舌面，称为瘀斑舌、瘀点舌（图 2-25，2-26，2-27）。

【临床意义】　主瘀血内阻。

【机理分析】　舌色泛现青紫或出现瘀斑是由肺失宣肃，或肝气不疏、血行不畅，或气虚无以推动血行而致血流障碍。

此外尚有暴力外伤，损伤血络，血液溢出而舌现斑点，舌色可无明显异常。舌色紫暗或舌上有斑点，多为瘀血内阻。

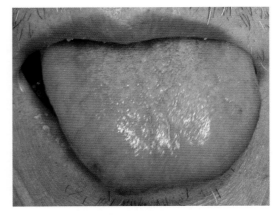

图 2-25　舌色红，舌前有瘀斑
（男　心绞痛）

A red tongue with ecchymosis on the anterior
of the tongue (male, angina pectoris)

5. 2 Purplish Red or Purplish Deep Red Tongue

Characteristics: A red tongue suffused with purple is a purplish red tongue (Diagram 2-23). A deep red tongue suffused with purple is a purplish deep red tongue (Diagram 2-24).

Clinical Significance: The blazing of heat toxin, and stagnation of Qi and Blood.

Pathogenesis Analysis: Tongue color that is a dull purple or purplish deep red, dry and withered with little fluid, scanty dry coating, is generally seen in heat syndromes, indicating the blazing of heat toxin, entering deep into the nutritive and blood levels, the nutritive Yin being scorched and the flow of Qi and Blood being obstructed.

5. 3 Tongue with Ecchymosis or Tongue with Purple Spots

Characteristics: A tongue partially covered with ecchymosis that varies in size, which does not protrude from the tongue surface, is labeled a tongue with ecchymoses or tongue with purple spots (Diagram 2-25、2-26、2-27).

Clinical Significance: Indicating an internal blood stasis.

Pathogenesis Analysis: Cyanosis of the tongue or tongue with ecchymoses due to impairment of the Lung's function of dispersing and descending, or the constraining of Liver Qi, sluggish flow of Blood, or Qi deficiency failing to transport Blood leading to obstructive Blood flow.

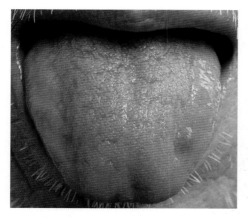

图 2-26 舌色鲜红，苔薄白，舌边有瘀点，
（男 上消化道出血）

A bright red tongue, a thin white coating, and purple spot on the tongue border (male, hemorrhage of the upper digestive tract)

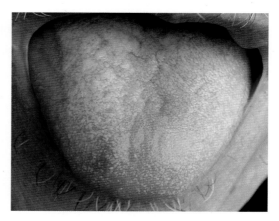

图 2-27 舌色淡红，舌前有瘀斑，苔淡黄腻
（男 高血压、脑梗塞）

A light red tongue, ecchymosis on the anterior of the tongue, and a pale yellow and greasy coating (male, hypertension, cerebral infarction)

Moreover a violent external injury will rupture blood vessels leading to the escape of blood into the surrounding tissue thus appearing as ecchymoses on the tongue without a change in color of the tongue. A dull purple tongue or a tongue with ecchymoses is generally indicative of internal blood stasis.

第三节　舌　　形

舌体的形质包括老嫩、胖瘦、点刺、裂纹等方面特征。分述如下：

一、老、嫩舌

舌质老嫩是舌色和形质的综合表现。根据舌质地的纹理及舌色的浅深，一般分为老舌、嫩舌两种。老和嫩是疾病虚实的标志之一。《辨舌指南·辨舌之神气》曰："凡舌质坚敛而苍老，不论苔色白、黄、灰、黑，病多属实；舌质浮胖兼娇嫩，不拘苔色灰、黑、黄、白，病多属虚。"

（一）老舌

【舌象特征】　舌质纹理粗糙或皱缩，舌体坚敛苍老，舌色较暗者为老舌（图2-28）。

【临床意义】　多见于实证。

【机理分析】　邪气亢盛、充斥体内，正气未衰，邪气壅滞于舌，故见舌质苍老。

（二）嫩舌

【舌象特征】　舌质纹理细腻，舌体浮胖娇嫩。舌色浅淡者为淡嫩舌（图2-29，2-30，2-31）；舌红而嫩为嫩红舌（图2-32，2-33）。

【临床意义】　嫩舌多见于虚证。气血不足，或阳气亏虚，精血不足。

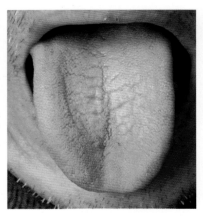

图2-28　舌色红，舌质苍老，舌面干燥，舌苔中部白腻厚并有裂纹（男　矽肺）

A red and rough tongue, with a dry tongue surface, and the central part of the tongue coating is thick, white and greasy with fissures (male, pneumoconiosis)

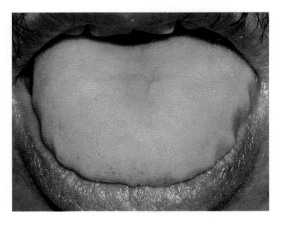

图2-29　舌色淡红，舌体胖嫩，舌边有齿痕，苔色白（男　肾病综合征）

A pale red tongue, with a puffy and tender tongue body, tooth-marked tongue borders, and a white coating (male, multiple fractures of the ribs)

SECTION THREE   TONGUE BODY SHAPE

The shapes of the tongue body can be described as rough and tender, swollen and thin, spotted and prickled, fissured etc. Aspects of these are detailed as follows:

1. Rough and Tender Tongue

A rough or tender tongue proper is the overall manifestation of tongue color and tongue body shape. According to the creases and color intensity of the tongue proper, it is generally separated into two groups: rough tongue and tender tongue. Rough and tender are one of the manifestations that mark the excessiveness or deficiency of a disease. *A Guide to Tongue Differentiation • Differentiating the Spirit of the Tongue* states: "All tongue proper that are stiff, restrained and appear aged, whether the coating color is white, yellow, gray or black, generally indicates an excess syndrome; if tongue proper is swollen and tender, whether coating color is gray, black, yellow, white, it is predominantly a deficiency syndrome."

1.1   Rough Tongue

Characteristics: A Rough tongue is where the creases of the tongue proper appear rough and coarse or wrinkly, the tongue body is stiff, restrained and looks aged, and the tongue color is dull (Diagram 2-28).

Clinical Significance: Generally seen in excess syndromes.

Pathogenesis Analysis: Hyperactivity of pathogenic Qi is abound within the body, the anti-pathogenic Qi is yet to decline, the pathogenic Qi is congested within the tongue hence the tongue proper appears aged.

1.2   Tender Tongue

Characteristics: The creases of the tongue proper appear fine and smooth, the tongue body is puffy and delicate. If the color of the tongue is light and pale, this is a pale and tender tongue (Diagram 2-29, 2-30, 2-31); if the tongue color is red and tender, this is a tender and red tongue (Diagram 2-32, 2-33).

Clinical Significance: The tender tongue is predominantly seen in deficiency syndromes. Qi and Blood deficiency, or Yang Qi deficiency, Essence and Blood deficiency.

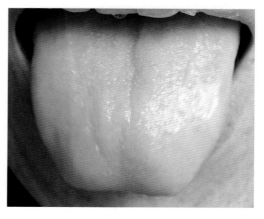

图 2-30 舌色淡，舌质嫩，苔薄
（男　末梢神经炎）

A pale and tender tongue, and a thin coating
(male, peripheral neuronitis)

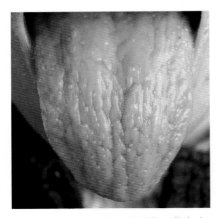

图 2-31　舌色淡红，舌质嫩，苔色白
（女　肾盂肾炎）

A pale red and tender tongue, and a white
coating (female, nephropyelitis)

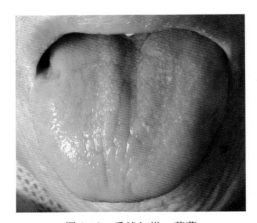

图 2-32　舌淡红嫩，苔薄
（女　肺癌骨转移）

A light red and tender tongue, and a thin coating
(female, lung cancer metastases to the bones)

【机理分析】　气血不足，无以上充于舌，或阳气亏虚，运血无力，则舌嫩色淡白。精血不足，则舌嫩红少苔。

二、胖、瘦舌

胖、瘦舌根据舌的形状、质地及其他伴随情况一般分为胖大舌、肿胀舌、瘦薄舌 3 种。

（一）胖大舌

【舌象特征】　舌体比正常的人大而厚，伸舌满口，称为胖大舌（图 2-34，2-35，2-36）。

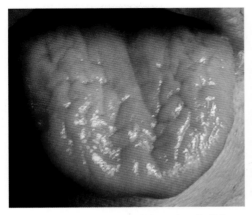

图 2-33　舌色红，舌质嫩，舌面有裂纹
（男　支气管炎）

A red and tender tongue, with fissures on the
tongue surface (male, bronchitis)

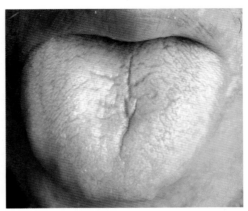

图 2-34　舌色淡，舌体胖大，舌苔淡黄
（男　左胸腔积液、左支气管病变、咳血）

A pale tongue, puffy and enlarged tongue body, and
a pale yellow tongue coating (male, hydropsy of the
left thoracic cavity, pathological change to the left
bronchus, coughing up blood)

Pathogenesis Analysis: Qi and Blood deficiency fails to ascend and nourish the tongue, or Yang Qi deficiency fails to transport Blood, leading to a pale and tender tongue. Essence and Blood deficiency resulting in a tender and red tongue with scanty coating.

2. Puffy And Thin Tongue

A puffy or thin tongue is classified according to the shape of the tongue, its proper, and other accompanying circumstances, generally into 3 groups: puffy tongue, swollen tongue, thin and emaciated tongue.

2.1 Puffy Tongue

Characteristics: A puffy tongue occurs when the tongue body is distended and larger than that of a normal tongue, and on extension of the tongue it can fill up the whole mouth (Diagram 2-34, 2-35, 2-36).

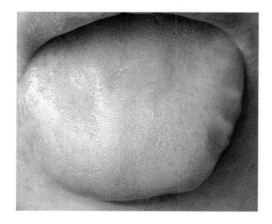

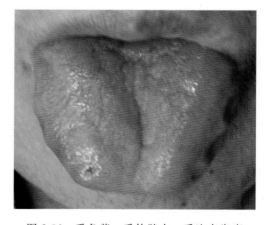

图 2-35 舌色淡，舌体胖大，边有齿痕，
苔浅黄（女 高血压）
A pale tongue, puffy and enlarged tongue body,
tooth-marked borders and a light yellow coating
(female, hypertension)

图 2-36 舌色紫，舌体胖大，舌边有齿痕
（男 多发性骨髓瘤）
Purple tongue, puffy and enlarged tongue
body, and tooth-marked tongue borders
(male, multiple myeloma)

【临床意义】　多主水湿内停。

【机理分析】　胖大舌多因脾肾阳虚、气化失常、津液输布障碍、体内水湿停滞所致。

胖大舌根据舌色、苔色、苔质等还可分为舌色淡白而胖大，舌淡白胖嫩、舌苔水滑，舌淡红或红而胖大、舌苔黄腻3种。

1. 舌色淡白而胖大

【舌象特征】　舌色淡白，舌体胖大（图2-37）。

【临床意义】　主气虚、阳虚。

【机理分析】　舌色淡白胖大多为气虚无以生血、无以推动血液和水液运行，阳虚则虚寒内生，水湿内停，故见舌色淡白胖大。

2. 舌淡白胖嫩、舌苔水滑

【舌象特征】　舌色淡白，舌体胖嫩，舌苔水滑（图2-38）。

【临床意义】　主阳虚水停。

【机理分析】　脾肾阳虚，津液不化，积水停饮。

3. 舌红而胖大

【舌象特征】　舌色淡红或红，舌体胖大，舌苔黄腻（图2-39，2-40）。

【临床意义】　主脾胃湿热。

【机理分析】　脾胃湿热或痰热内蕴，湿热痰饮上溢所致。

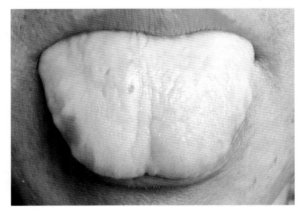

图 2-37　舌色淡白，舌体胖大，舌边有齿痕，苔淡黄厚
（男　慢性肾功能衰竭、高钾血症）
A pale white tongue, puffy and enlarged tongue body, tooth-marked tongue borders, and thick yellow coating (male, chronic renal failure, hyperkalemia)

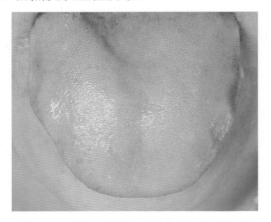

图 2-38　舌淡白胖嫩，边有齿痕，舌苔水滑
（女　血小板减少症）
A pale white, puffy and tender tongue, tooth-marked borders, and a watery and slippery tongue coating (female, thrombocytopenia)

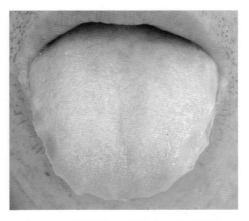

图 2-39　舌色淡红，舌胖大，边有齿痕，苔中根黄（男　原发性支气管肺癌）
A light red tongue that is puffy and enlarged, tooth-marked borders, and the center and root of the coating is yellow (male, primary bronchogenic carcinoma)

Clinical Significance: Generally indicates an interior retention of damp-water syndrome.

Pathogenesis Analysis: A puffy tongue is mostly due to the deficiency of Spleen Yang and Kidney Yang, dysfunction of Qi transformation, obstruction to the distribution of body fluids, leading to the retention of dampness and water in the interior.

A puffy tongue is classified according to the colors of the tongue body and coating, the proper of coating generally into 3 groups, pale white and puffy tongue, pale white, puffy and tender tongue with a moist and slippery coating, pale red or red and puffy tongue with a yellow and greasy coating.

2.1.1 Pale White and Puffy Tongue

Characteristics: Tongue color is pale white and tongue body is puffy (Diagram 2-37).

Clinical Significance: Signifying Qi deficiency, Yang deficiency.

Pathogenesis Analysis: A pale white and enlarged tongue is chiefly due to the deficiency of Qi unable to produce Blood, failing to transport Blood and fluids. Yang deficiency leads to internal deficiency cold and dampness stagnation in the body hence the tongue appears pale, white and enlarged.

2.1.2 Pale White, Puffy and Tender Tongue with a Moist and Slippery Coating

Characteristics: Tongue color is pale white, tongue body is puffy and tender, and tongue coating is moist and slippery (Diagram 2-38).

Clinical Significance: Indicating Yang deficiency and retention of water.

Pathogenesis Analysis: Spleen Yang and Kidney Yang deficiency failing to transform water, leading to the accumulation and retention of water and fluids.

2.1.3 Red and Puffy Tongue

Characteristics: Tongue color is pale red or red, tongue body is puffy, and tongue coating is yellow and greasy (Diagram 2-39, 2-40).

Clinical Significance: Indicating damp heat in the Stomach and Spleen.

Pathogenesis Analysis: Caused by damp heat in the Stomach and Spleen or accumulation of phlegm heat in the interior, damp heat and phlegm fluid overflowing to the tongue.

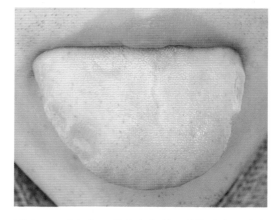

图 2-40 舌色红，舌尖有芒刺，舌体胖大，舌边
有齿痕，舌苔黄腻（男 上呼吸道感染）

A red tongue, with prickles on the tongue tip, puffy
and enlarged tongue body, tooth-marked tongue
borders, and a yellow and greasy tongue coating
(male, upper respiratory tract infection)

（二）肿胀舌

【舌象特征】 舌体胀大满嘴，舌色鲜红或青紫，甚则舌肿胀而不能收缩回口中（图 2-41）。

【临床意义】 多主心脾热盛、外感湿热。

【机理分析】 舌胀大而色红者多为里热。

肿胀舌根据舌色的不同还可进一步划分为舌肿胀色红绛、舌紫而肿胀 2 种。

1. 舌肿胀色红绛

【舌象特征】 舌体肿胀，舌色红绛（图 2-42）。

【临床意义】 主心脾热盛。

【机理分析】 舌肿胀色红绛，多见于心脾热盛，热毒上壅。

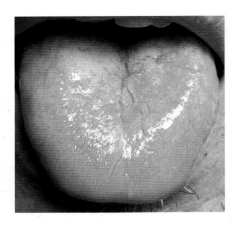 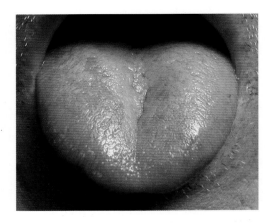

图 2-41 舌色红，舌体肿胀，前部少苔，根部苔黄腻（男 慢性肾小球肾炎）

A red and swollen tongue, with scanty coating on the anterior of the tongue, and yellow and greasy coating at the root (male, chronic glomerular nephritis)

图 2-42 舌色红绛肿胀，舌尖有芒刺，舌苔前部剥落，根部色淡黄灰腻（男 慢性肾功能衰竭）

A deep red and swollen tongue, prickles on the tongue tip, peeled anterior coating, and at the root the coating is grayish yellow and greasy (male, chronic renal failure)

2. 舌紫而肿胀

【舌象特征】 舌色紫，舌体肿胀（图 2-43，2-44）。

【临床意义】 主邪热夹酒毒上壅。

【机理分析】 邪热夹酒毒上壅，充斥血络，可见舌色紫，舌体肿胀。先天性舌血管瘤患者，可见舌的局部肿胀色紫，属于血络瘀阻的局部病变，多无全身辨证意义。

2.2 Swollen Tongue

Characteristics: Tongue body is swollen and fills the mouth, tongue color is either bright red or cyanosis. In extreme cases, the tongue is so swollen that the tongue is unable to retract back into the mouth (Diagram 2-41).

Clinical Significance: Signifying abundance of heat in the Heart and Spleen, and the external contraction of damp heat.

Pathogenesis Analysis: A swollen tongue that is red in color is generally indicative of an interior heat syndrome.

Swollen tongues are classified according to the colours of the tongue generally into 2 groups: a swollen and deep red tongue, or a purple and swollen tongue.

2.2.1 Swollen and Deep Red Tongue

Characteristics: Tongue body is swollen and tongue color is deep red (Diagram 2-42).

Clinical Significance: Indicating abundance of heat in the Heart and Spleen.

Pathogenesis Analysis: A swollen tongue that is deep red in color is generally seen in the abundance of heat in the Heart and Spleen, or heat toxin accumulating in the upper.

2.2.2 Purple and Swollen Tongue

Characteristics: Tongue color is purple and tongue body is swollen (Diagram 2-43, 2-44).

Clinical Significance: Indicating pathogenic heat and alcoholic toxin accumulating in the upper.

Pathogenesis Analysis: Pathogenic heat and alcoholic toxin accumulating in the upper and flooding the blood vessels can appear as a purple tongue and a swollen tongue body. In congenital hemangioma (benign tumor made up of blood vessels) sufferers, there can be partial swelling and purple coloring of the tongue, a localized pathological change indicating blood stasis in the blood vessels, predominantly no significance in showing the whole condition of the body.

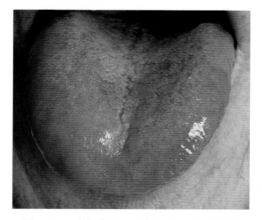

图 2-43 舌色紫红，舌体肿胀，舌苔根部
淡黄腻（男 原发性支气管肺癌）
A purplish red and swollen tongue, and a pale yellow and greasy tongue coating at the root (male, primary bronchogenic carcinoma)

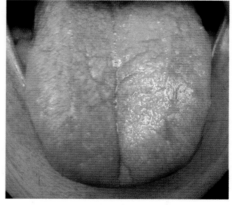

图 2-44 舌色暗红，舌体肿胀，舌苔根部
淡黄腐腻（男 胸腔积液待查）
A dull red and swollen tongue, and a pale yellow, greasy and curdy tongue coating at the root (male, hydropsy of the thoracic cavity awaiting examination)

（三）瘦薄舌

【舌象特征】 舌体比正常舌瘦小而薄，称为瘦薄舌（图 2-45，2-46）。

【临床意义】 多主气血不足、阴虚火旺。

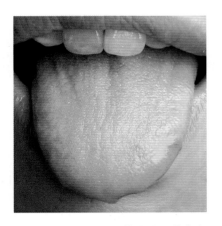 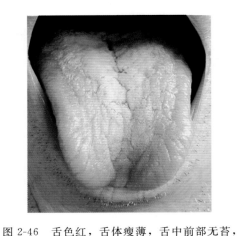

图 2-45 舌色暗，舌体瘦小，苔薄白
（女 慢性支气管炎急性发作）
A dull tongue，the tongue body is small and emaciated，and a thin white coating (female，acute attack of chronic bronchitis)

图 2-46 舌色红，舌体瘦薄，舌中前部无苔，
根部淡黄厚腐腻（男 慢性阻塞性肺病）
A red tongue，thin and emaciated tongue body，absence of coating at the center and anterior of the tongue，a pale yellow thick，curdy and greasy coating at the root (male，chronic obstructive pulmonary disease)

【机理分析】 瘦薄舌总由气血阴液不足，舌失濡养所致。

根据舌形和舌色的改变，瘦薄舌可分为舌瘦薄而红绛、舌瘦薄而淡 2 种。

1. 舌瘦薄而红绛

【舌象特征】 舌体瘦薄，舌色红绛（图 2-47）。

【临床意义】 主阴虚火旺。

【机理分析】 多见于阴虚火旺，阴液亏虚无以滋养舌体，故舌瘦薄，阴虚火旺则舌色红绛，阴液不能上承则舌干少苔或无苔。

2. 舌瘦薄而淡

【舌象特征】 舌体瘦薄，舌色淡（图 2-48）。

【临床意义】 主气血两虚。

【机理分析】 多见于久病气血两虚，血不上荣。

2.3 Thin and Emaciated Tongue

Characteristics: A thin and emaciated tongue in comparison to a normal tongue is thinner and appears emaciated (Diagram 2-45, 2-46).

Clinical Significance: Indicating Qi and Blood deficiency, Yin deficiency with up-flaming of fire.

Pathogenesis Analysis: A thin and emaciated tongue is chiefly due to the deficiency of Qi, Blood, Yin and fluids failing to nourish the tongue.

Thin and emaciated tongues are classified according to the shapes and colours of the tongue body, generally into 2 groups: thin and deep red tongue and thin and pale tongue.

2.3.1 Thin and Deep Red Tongue

Characteristics: Tongue body is thin and emaciated, and the tongue color is deep red (Diagram 2-47).

Clinical Significance: Indicating Yin deficiency with up-flaming of fire.

Pathogenesis Analysis: Generally seen in Yin deficiency with up-flaming of fire, where Yin fluids are deficient thus fails to nourish the tongue body therefore appearing thin and emaciated. Yin deficiency with up-flaming of fire causing the deep red color of the tongue, the Yin fluids cannot ascend causing a dry tongue with scanty or no coating.

2.3.2 Thin and Pale Tongue

Characteristics: Tongue body is thin and emaciated, and tongue color is pale (Diagram 2-48).

Clinical Significance: Indicating Qi and Blood deficiency.

Pathogenesis Analysis: Generally seen in chronic diseases where Qi and Blood are deficient thus Blood fails to nourish the tongue.

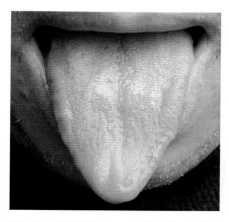

图 2-47 舌色两边红，舌体瘦薄，苔薄黄
（男 肺炎）

Red tongue borders, thin and emaciated tongue body, and a thin yellow coating (male, pneumonia)

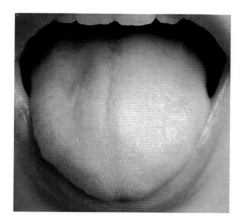

图 2-48 舌色淡，舌体瘦小，苔中根淡黄
（男 再生障碍性贫血）

A pale tongue, small and emaciated tongue body, and a pale yellow coating at the center and root
（male, aplastic anemia）

三、点、刺舌

点刺是指蕈状乳头肿胀或高突的病理特征。

【舌象特征】 点指突起于舌面的红色或紫红色的星点，大者称星，小者称点（图 2-49）。刺，是指蕈状乳头增大、高突，并形成尖峰，形如芒刺，抚之棘手，为芒刺舌（图 2-50，2-51）。

根据点刺出现的部位，可区分热在何脏。如舌尖生点刺，为心火亢盛（图2-52）；舌中生点刺，为胃肠热盛（图 2-53）；舌两边生点刺，为肝胆火热（图 2-54）。

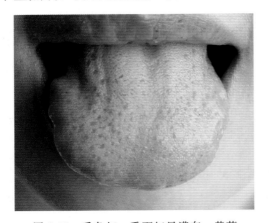

图 2-49　舌色红，舌面红星满布，黄苔
（女　急性肝炎）

A red tongue, with red stars distributed all over, and a yellow coating (female, acute hepatitis)

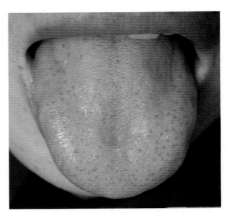

图 2-50　舌色红，舌边尖有芒刺，舌苔黄
（女　大叶性肺炎）

A red tongue, with prickles on the tongue borders and tip, and a yellow tongue coating (female, chronic gastritis)

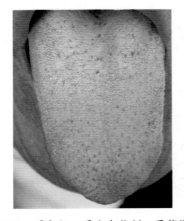

图 2-51　舌色红，舌尖有芒刺，舌苔根厚
（男　高血压病）

A red tongue, with prickles on the tongue tip, and a thick coating at the root (male, hypertension)

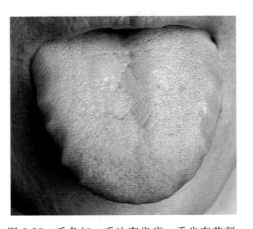

图 2-52　舌色红，舌边有齿痕，舌尖有芒刺，舌苔淡黄腻（男　冠状动脉粥样硬化性心脏病）

A red tongue, with tooth-marked tongue borders, prickles on the tongue tip, and a pale yellow and greasy tongue coating (male, coronary artherosclotic heart disease)

3. Spots and Prickles Tongue

Spots and prickles are the result of pathological changes in the fungiform papillae that become swollen or due to its elevated protrusion.

Characteristics: Spots refer to the protrusions on the surface of the tongue that are red or purplish red in color. The larger ones are named stars while the smaller ones are simply called spots (Diagram 2-49). Prickles are formed when the fungiform papillae on the tongue are bigger than normal, the protrusions are higher with a pointed apex, shaped like prickles. On touching or stroking of the tongue it will feel thorny, thus being a prickled tongue (Diagram 2-50, 2-51).

According to the location of the spots and prickles, it can be distinguished within which organ there is heat.

Prickles on the tip of the tongue indicate exuberance of Heart fire (Diagram 2-52).

Prickles on the center of the tongue indicate exuberance of heat in the Stomach and Intestines (Diagram 2-53).

Prickles on the borders of the tongue indicate exuberance of heat in the Liver and Gall Bladder (Diagram 2-54).

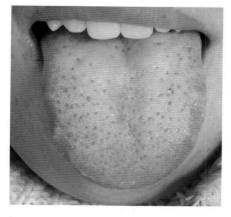

图 2-53 舌色红，舌前中部红点，苔白腻
（女 慢性支气管炎急性发作）
A red tongue, red spots on the anterior and centre of the tongue, and a greasy white coating (female, acute attack of chronic bronchitis)

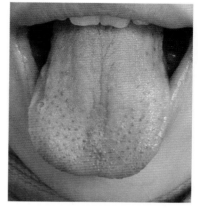

图 2-54 舌色红，舌尖边有芒刺，舌苔灰黄厚腻
（女 冠状动脉粥样硬化性心脏病）
A red tongue, prickles on the tongue tip and borders, and a thick grayish yellow and greasy coating (female, coronary artherosclerotic heart disease)

【临床意义】 提示脏腑阳热亢盛，或为血分热盛。

【机理分析】 点刺是蕈状乳头肿胀或比正常高突的病理特征。点，是蕈状乳头体积增大，数目增多，乳头内充血水肿，甚至形成尖峰，形如芒刺，多为邪热内蕴、充斥舌络。点刺数目的多少与邪热程度有关，点刺越多，邪热越盛。

观察点刺的颜色，可以估计气血运行情况以及疾病的程度。如点刺鲜红为血热内盛，或阴虚火旺；点刺色绛紫为热盛而气血壅滞。

四、裂纹舌

【舌象特征】 舌面上出现各种形状的裂纹、裂沟，深浅不一，多少不等，统称为裂纹舌。

裂纹可呈现"人""｜""井"等形状，严重者可呈脑回状、卵石状，或如刀割、剪碎一样（图 2-55，2-56，2-57，2-58，2-59，2-60，2-61，2-62）。

【临床意义】 多由精血亏虚，或阴虚火旺、脾虚湿浸所致。

【机理分析】 裂纹舌多由舌体失养，舌面乳头萎缩或组织皲裂所致。是全身营养不良的一种表现。

裂纹舌根据其形状，裂纹多少、浅深及伴随的舌色不同，又可分为舌色淡白而裂、舌色红绛而裂、全舌绛色或有横直裂纹而短小、舌色淡白胖嫩边有齿痕又兼见裂纹、先天性裂纹舌等。

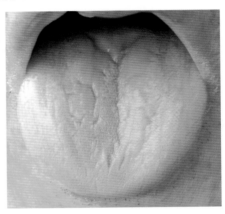

图 2-55 舌色红，舌面有"人"字形裂纹，舌面少苔（男　冠状动脉粥样硬化性心脏病）
A red tongue, with a "人" shaped fissure on the tongue surface, and scanty coating (male, coronary artherosclerotic heart disease)

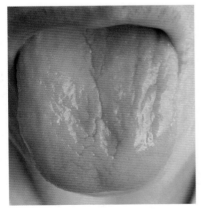

图 2-56 舌色红，舌面无苔，伴有"人"字形细小裂纹（女　药疹、高血压）
A red tongue, absence of coating, with a "人" shaped fissure that is very small (female, medicinal exanthema, Hypertension)

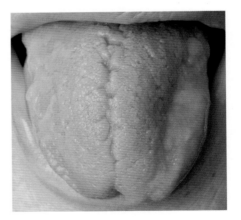

图 2-57 舌色红，舌中有深如刀割纵形裂纹（女　腹痛待查）
A red tongue, down the midline of the tongue is a deep vertical fissure like a cut from a knife (female, lumbago awaiting examination)

Clinical Significance: Indicating the exuberance of heat in the internal organs, or exuberance of heat in the Blood level.

Pathogenesis Analysis: The spots and prickles refer to the pathological characteristics of the fungiform papillae that are swollen or protruding higher than normal. Spots are the enlargement and increase in number of fungiform papillae, the heads of the papillae are filled with blood and there is edema, even to the point where the peak is pointed, and shaped like prickles, predominantly being the internal accumulation of pathogenic heat reaching up to the collaterals of the tongue. The more the spots and prickles, the more exuberant the pathogenic heat.

Examining the color of the spots and prickles can assist in determining the condition of the transportation of Qi and Blood and the severity of a disease. For example, if spots and prickles are bright red in color, this indicates the internal accumulation of heat in the blood or Yin deficiency with up-flaming of fire; if spots and prickles are a purplish and deep red color, it is indicative of a superabundance of heat with accumulation of Qi and Blood.

4. Fissured Tongue

Characteristics: Fissures and grooves that appear on the tongue can come in a variety of shapes, that vary in depth or shallowness, that differ in numbers, these are all labeled as a fissured tongue. The fissures can take on shapes of "人", "|", "井" etc, and in extreme cases can appear in forms like brain fissures, pebbles, or like it's been cut to shreds with a knife (Diagrams2-55,2-56,2-57,2-58,2-59,2-60,2-61,2-62).

Clinical Significance: Mostly due to Essence and Blood deficiency, or Yin deficiency with up-flaming of fire, Spleen deficiency with retention of damp.

Pathogenesis Analysis: Fissured tongues are predominantly the result of the tongue body failing to be nourished, the papillae on the surface of the tongue are shriveled or the tissues on the tongue are chapped. This is a sign that the nourishment of the whole body is poor.

A fissured tongue can be subdivided in accordance with its shape, the quantity of the fissures, their intensity of tongue color, generally into pale white and fissured tongue, deep red and fissured tongue, tongue completely deep red or with horizontal straight and short fissures, pale white enlarged and tender tongue with fissures and teeth-marked borders, and congenital fissured tongue etc.

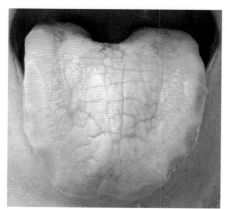

图 2-58　舌色淡红，舌面裂纹呈井字形，舌边
有齿痕（男　2 型糖尿病、糖尿病肾病）
A pale red tongue, with "井" shaped fissures on the
tongue surface and tooth-marked tongue borders
(male, type Ⅱ diabetes, diabetic nephropathy)

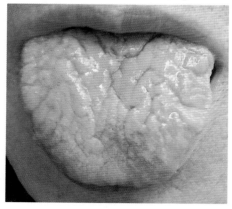

图 2-59　舌色嫩红，舌面裂纹形似猪脑，
苔黄腻（男　不稳定型心绞痛）
A red and tender tongue, pig's brain-like fissures
on the tongue surface, and a yellow and greasy
coating (male, unstable angina pectoris)

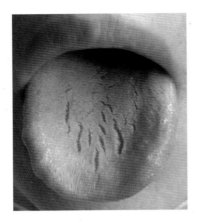

图 2-60 舌色红，舌面裂纹深如刀割，
苔色黄（女 糖尿病）

A red tongue, deep fissures similar to
cuts from a knife on the tongue surface,
and a yellow coating (female, diabetes)

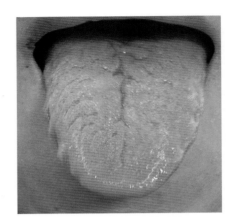

图 2-61 舌嫩红，裂纹满布，
边有齿痕（男 便秘待查）

A tender and red tongue, fissures distributed
all over, and tooth-marked borders (male,
constipation awaiting examination)

（一）舌色淡白而裂

【舌象特征】 舌色淡白而裂（图 2-63）。

【临床意义】 血虚之候。

【机理分析】 多为血虚，血不上荣于舌所致。故《辨舌指南·辨舌之质本》认为："有纹者血衰也。纹少、纹浅者衰之微；纹多、纹深者衰之甚也。"

（二）舌色红绛而有裂纹

【舌象特征】 舌色红绛而裂（图 2-64）。

【临床意义】 热盛伤津，或阴虚火旺。

【机理分析】 多由热盛伤津，或阴虚火旺、阴津耗损、舌失濡养所致。

（三）全舌绛色，或有横直裂纹而短小

【舌象特征】 全舌绛色，或有横直裂纹而短小（图 2-65）。

【临床意义】 阴虚液涸。

【机理分析】 表明阴虚液涸，舌体失养。

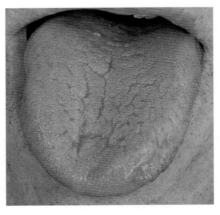

图 2-62 舌色暗红，舌质坚敛苍老，
舌面裂纹深如刀割（男 肝硬化）

A dull red tongue, stiff, restrained and
rough, and fissures as deep as knife cuts
(male, cirrhosis of the liver)

4.1   Pale White and Fissured Tongue

Characteristics: Tongue color is pale white with fissures (Diagram 2-63).

Clinical Significance: The manifestation of Blood deficiency.

Pathogenesis Analysis: Generally signifying Blood deficiency where Blood cannot ascend to nourish the tongue. Thus *Guide to Tongue Differentiation • Differentiating Tongue Propers* acknowledges: "A cracked tongue indicates exhaustion of Blood. The fewer and more superficial the cracks, the milder the disease. The deeper and more numerous the cracks, the more serious the disease. "

4.2   Deep Red and Fissured Tongue

Characteristics: Tongue color is deep red with fissures (Diagram 2-64).

Clinical Significance: Indicating the exuberance of heat consuming the fluids, or Yin deficiency with up-flaming of fire.

Pathogenesis Analysis: Chiefly due to exuberant heat injuring the fluids, or Yin deficiency with up-flaming of fire. Yin fluids are consumed, thus failing to nourish the tongue.

4.3   Tongue Completely Deep Red or with Horizontal, Straight and Short Fissures

Characteristics: The entire tongue is deep red in color, or with horizontal, straight and short fissures (Diagram 2-65).

Clinical Significance: Yin deficiency consuming the fluids.

Pathogenesis Analysis: Indicating that Yin deficiency has consumed the fluids thus unable to nourish the tongue.

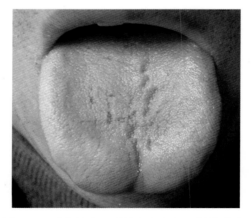

图 2-63　舌色淡白，舌前中部有似刀割样裂纹，
舌苔色黄腻（男　消化性溃疡伴大出血）
A pale white tongue, with fissures on the anterior
and centre of the tongue similar to cuts from a knife,
and a greasy yellow tongue coating (male, massive
hemorrhaging from a peptic ulcer)

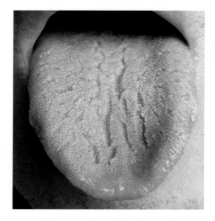

图 2-64　舌色红，舌面较深裂纹，苔根淡黄厚
（男　慢粒细胞性白血病急变）
A red tongue, with relatively deep fissures
on the tongue surface, the coating at the root
is thick and yellow (male, acute change in
chronic granulocytic leukemia)

（四）舌色淡白胖嫩边有齿痕又兼见裂纹

【舌象特征】 舌色淡白胖嫩，边有齿痕，又兼见裂纹（图2-66）。

【临床意义】 血虚，或脾虚湿侵。

【机理分析】 因脾失健运、湿邪内蕴、浸淫舌体、舌失气血濡养所致。

在健康人中大约有0.5%的人在舌面上有纵、横深沟，裂纹中有苔覆盖，且无不适症状，为先天性舌裂，必须与病理性裂纹舌作鉴别（图2-67）。

五、齿痕舌

【舌象特征】 舌边缘有牙齿压迫的痕迹，多伴舌体胖大（图2-68，2-69）。

【临床意义】 主脾虚、水湿内盛证。

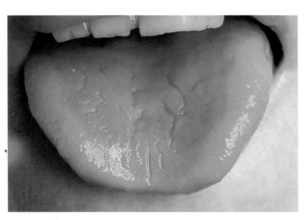

图2-65 舌色绛，舌面有裂纹，无苔
（女 发热原因待查）
A deep red tongue, with fissures on the tongue surface, and an absence of coating (female, cause of fever awaiting examination)

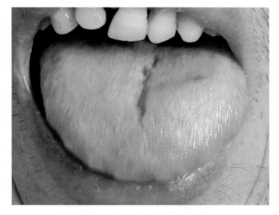

图2-66 舌色淡紫，舌边有齿痕，中有裂纹，苔淡黄根稍厚（男 高血压病、冠状动脉粥样硬化性心脏病）
A pale purple tongue, tooth-marked tongue borders, fissure down the midline, and a pale yellow coating that is slightly thicker at the root (male, hypertension, coronary artheroslcerotic heart disease)

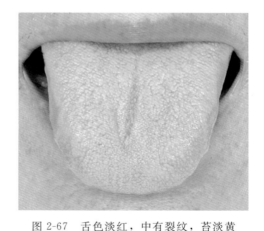

图2-67 舌色淡红，中有裂纹，苔淡黄
（男 健康人）
A pale red tongue, with a fissure down the midline, and a pale yellow coating (male, healthy individual)

【机理分析】 舌边有齿痕，多因舌体胖大受牙齿挤压所致，故多与胖大舌同见。舌体不胖大而出现齿痕，是舌质娇嫩的齿痕舌。

此外，有先天性齿痕舌者，多见舌体不大，舌淡红而嫩，边有轻微齿痕；病中见之表明病情较轻，常见于小儿及气血不足患者。

4.4 Pale White, Enlarged and Tender Tongue with Fissures, and Teeth Marks on the Borders

Characteristics: The tongue is pale white, enlarged and tender with fissures, and teeth marks on the borders (Diagram 2-66).

Clinical Significance: Blood deficiency, or Spleen deficiency with retention of damp.

Pathogenesis Analysis: Chiefly due to Spleen deficiency with retention of damp. Due to the failure of Spleen in transportation, the accumulation of pathogenic damp in the interior, seeping to the tongue body, Qi and Blood fails to nourish the tongue.

Among healthy individuals there are approximately 0.5% that have deep grooves that are vertical or horizontal, and fissures covered by coating, yet there is an absence of other indisposed signs or symptoms, thus belonging to congenital fissured tongue and it is vital to differentiate this with a pathological fissured tongue (Diagram 2-67).

5. Tooth-marked Tongue

Characteristics: The borders of the tongue are indented with tooth-marks, generally accompanied by an enlargement of the tongue (Diagram 2-68, 2-69).

Clinical Significance: Indicating Spleen deficiency and internal retention of dampness.

Pathogenesis Analysis: The tooth-marks on the sides of the tongue are chiefly due to the enlargement of the tongue body being pressed against the teeth, thus a tooth-marked tongue is commonly seen together with an enlarged tongue. A tongue that is not enlarged yet tooth-marked is a tender and tooth-marked tongue.

Furthermore, there are congenital tooth-marked tongues where the tongue is light red and tender yet not enlarged, and the borders of the tongue have slight tooth-marks. When tooth-marks are present during a disease, it indicates that the disease is mild. It is commonly seen in children and those with Qi and Blood deficiency.

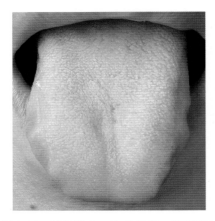

图 2-68 舌色淡白，边有齿痕，舌苔薄白
（男　自身免疫性溶血性贫血）
A pale white tongue, with tooth-marked borders, and a thin white tongue coating
（male, autoimmune hemolytic anemia）

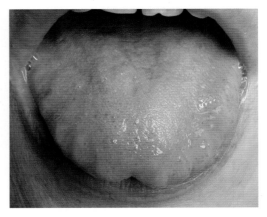

图 2-69 舌色暗红，舌边有齿痕，苔灰黄腻
（女　气胸）
A dull red tongue, with tooth-marked tongue borders, and a greasy grayish yellow coating
（female, pneumothorax）

齿痕舌根据所伴随的舌色、舌形情况一般分为舌淡胖大有齿痕、舌色淡红有齿痕、舌红肿胀有齿痕3种。

（一）舌淡有齿痕

【舌象特征】 舌淡胖大而润，舌边有齿痕者（图2-70，2-71，2-72）。

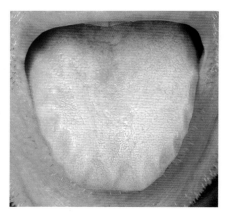

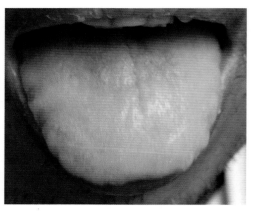

图2-70 舌色淡，舌体胖大，边有齿痕，苔薄
（男 巨幼红细胞性贫血）
A pale, puffy and enlarged tongue with tooth-marked borders, and a thin coating (male, megaloblastic anemia)

图2-71 舌色淡，舌边有齿痕，苔灰黑
（男 重度贫血）
A pale tongue, tooth-marked tongue borders and a grayish black coating (male, severe anemia)

【临床意义】 多为寒湿壅盛，或阳虚水停而致。

【机理分析】 寒湿壅盛或阳虚水停使舌体经脉收引，舌体失养，故舌色偏淡，水湿浸淫，故舌体胖大。

（二）舌色淡红有齿痕

【舌象特征】 舌色淡红，舌边有齿痕（图2-73）。

【临床意义】 见于脾虚、气虚；亦可为先天性齿痕舌。

【机理分析】 脾虚、气虚水湿运化失常，舌体胖大压迫齿缘，故见之。

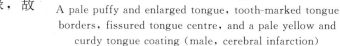

图2-72 舌色淡，舌体胖大，舌边齿痕，舌中裂，舌苔淡黄而腐（男 脑梗塞）
A pale puffy and enlarged tongue, tooth-marked tongue borders, fissured tongue centre, and a pale yellow and curdy tongue coating (male, cerebral infarction)

（三）舌红肿胀有齿痕

【舌象特征】 舌红肿胀满口，舌边有齿痕（图2-74，2-75）。

【临床意义】 湿热痰浊之证。

Tooth-marked tongues are divided according to the tongue color and tongue shape, generally into 3 types: pale enlarged and tooth-marked tongue, pale red and tooth-marked tongue, red swollen and tooth-marked tongue.

5.1 Pale Tooth-marked Tongue

Characteristics: The tongue is pale, enlarged and moist, and the borders of the tongue are tooth-marked (Diagram 2-70,2-71,2-72).

Clinical Significance: Indicates the internal stagnation of damp cold, or Yang deficiency with the retention of dampness.

Pathogenesis Analysis: Internal stagnation of damp cold or Yang deficiency with the retention of dampness causes the meridians of the tongue body to contract, the tongue body fails to be nourished, thus the tongue color tends to be pale. The accumulation of dampness and fluids results in the enlargement of the tongue body.

5.2 Light Red and Tooth-marked Tongue

Characteristics: Tongue color is light red, and the sides of the tongue are tooth-marked (Diagram 2-73).

Clinical Significance: Seen in Spleen deficiency, Qi deficiency; or belong to a congenital tooth-marked tongue.

Pathogenesis Analysis: Spleen deficiency and Qi deficiency causes a disharmony in the transformation and transportation of dampness and fluids, the tongue body becomes enlarged and is pressed against the edges of the teeth, thus a tooth-marked tongue is seen.

5.3 Red and Swollen Tooth-marked Tongue

Characteristics: The tongue is red and swollen so that it fills up the mouth, with tooth-marks on the sides of the tongue (Diagram 2-74, 2-75).

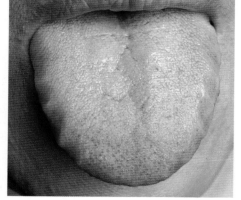

图 2-73 舌色淡红，舌边有齿痕，舌尖有芒刺，
舌苔淡黄腻（男 冠状动脉粥样硬化性心脏病）
A light red tongue, tooth-marked tongue borders, prickles on the tongue tip, and a pale yellow and greasy tongue coating (male, coronary artherosclerotic heart disease)

Clinical Significance: Indicates a syndrome of damp heat and turbid phlegm.

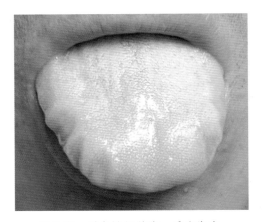

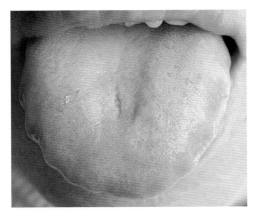

图 2-74 舌色淡红肿胀，舌边齿痕，
苔色淡黄（男 33 慢性腹泻）
A light red and swollen tongue, tooth-marked
borders, and a pale yellow coating
（male, 33 chronic diarrhea）

图 2-75 舌色红，舌体肿胀，边有齿痕，
苔色薄黄（女 冠状动脉粥样硬化性心脏病）
A red and swollen tongue, tooth-marked
borders, and a thin yellow coating（female,
coronary artherosclerotic heart disease）

【机理分析】 为湿热痰浊内蕴，充斥舌体脉络。

第四节 舌 的 动 态

舌的动态，又称舌态。舌体活动灵便，伸缩自如，为正常舌态，提示气血充盛，经脉通调，脏腑健旺。常见的病理舌态有舌体痿软、强硬、震颤、歪斜、吐弄和短缩等异常变化。

一、痿软舌

【舌象特征】 舌体软弱无力，不能随意伸缩回旋者，称为痿软舌（图 2-76）。

【临床意义】 多为伤阴或气血俱虚。

【机理分析】 痿软舌多因气血亏虚、阴液损伤，无以濡养舌肌与舌脉，致使舌体痿软。

痿软舌一般分为舌痿软而红绛少苔、舌痿软而舌色枯白无华2 种。

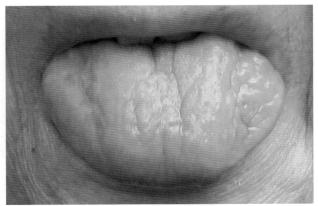

图 2-76 舌色红，舌体胖大而痿软，舌面无苔
（男 胃癌）
A red. puffy, enlarged and flaccid tongue, and
an absent tongue coating（male, stomach cancer）

（一）舌痿软而红绛少苔

【舌象特征】 舌痿软而红绛少苔（图 2-77）。

Pathogenesis Analysis: Due to the internal accumulation of damp heat with turbid phlegm flooding to the collaterals of the tongue.

SECTION FOUR MOVEMENT OF THE TONGUE

The normal movement of a tongue is one that is flexible and nimble, that extends and retracts smoothly, indicating the sufficiency of Qi and Blood, the harmonious circulation of the meridians and vessels, and the prosperous health of the internal organs. The common pathological changes in the movement of a tongue include flaccid, stiff, quivering, deviated, protruding and wagging, short and shrunken etc.

1. Flaccid Tongue

Characteristics: The tongue is flabby and weak, and unable to extend and retract (Diagram 2-76).

Clinical significance: Indicating consumption of Yin or the deficiency of Qi and Blood.

Pathogenesis Analysis: Predominantly due to the deficiency of Qi and Blood, and the consumption of Yin and fluids, failing to nourish the muscle and veins of the tongue, causing the flaccidity of the tongue body.

A flaccid tongue is generally categorized into 2 types, as a flaccid and deep red tongue with scanty coating, and a flaccid and ashen white tongue lacking vitality.

1.1 Flaccid and Deep Red Tongue with Scanty Coating

Characteristics: The tongue is flaccid and deep red in color with scanty coating (Diagram 2-77).

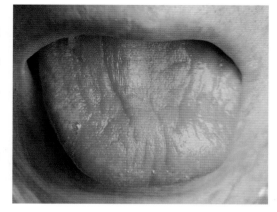

图 2-77 舌色红绛，舌萎软而少苔
（男 胰腺癌）
A deep red and flaccid tongue, with scanty coating (male, pancreatic cancer)

【临床意义】 多主邪热伤阴，或阴虚已极。

【机理分析】 多见于外感热病后期，邪热伤阴，或内伤久病，阴虚火旺。新病舌干红而痿，主热病津伤；舌红干而渐痿者，是肝肾阴亏已极之象。

（二）舌痿软而舌色枯白无华

【舌象特征】 舌痿软而舌色枯白无华（图 2-78）。

【临床意义】 属于气血俱虚。

【机理分析】 多因久病气血虚衰，舌体失养所致。

二、强硬舌

【舌象特征】 舌失柔和，屈伸不利，或板硬强直，不能转动者，称为强硬舌（图 2-79）。

【临床意义】 多见于热入心包，或为高热伤津，或为风痰阻络。

【机理分析】《千金要方·七窍病上》指出："舌强不能言，病在脏腑。"说明舌强硬一般不是局部病变，而是关系到内脏的病变。强硬舌可见于外感热病、热入心包、心神受扰、舌无所主；或高热伤津、筋脉失养、舌体失柔所致；或肝风夹痰、风痰阻络、肝阳上亢、筋脉失养，而致舌体强硬不能转动。

强硬舌根据舌色及舌苔情况一般分为舌强硬而舌色红绛少津、舌强硬而舌苔厚腻等。

（一）舌强硬而舌色红绛少津

【舌象特征】 舌体强硬，舌色红绛少津（图 2-80）。

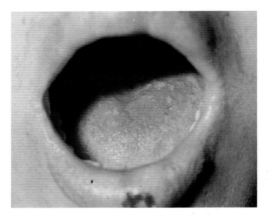

图 2-78 舌色枯白无华，舌体萎软（女 胃癌）
An ashen white tongue without vitality, and a flaccid tongue body (female, stomach cancer)

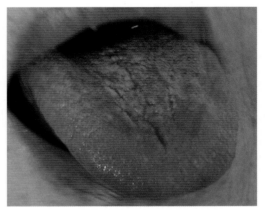

图 2-79 舌色紫暗，舌体强硬，舌面有裂纹，舌苔淡黄而腐腻（女 脑梗塞）
A dull purple tongue, stiff tongue body, fissures on the tongue surface, and a pale yellow, greasy and curdy tongue coating (female, cerebral infarction)

Clinical significance: Seen when pathogenic heat consumes Yin or the extreme exhaustion of Yin.

Pathogenesis Analysis: Chiefly seen in the later stages of an externally contracted febrile disease, pathogenic heat injures Yin, or internal impairment due to chronic disease, Yin deficiency and exuberance of fire. In an acute disease, the tongue is dry, red and flaccid indicating consumption of fluids due to febrile disease; a tongue that is red, dry and increasingly flaccid indicates the extreme exhaustion of Liver Yin and Kidney Yin.

1.2   Flaccid and Dull White Tongue Lacking Vitality

Characteristics: The tongue is flaccid and dull white in color that is lacking vitality (Diagram 2-78).

Clinical significance: Pertaining to the deficiency of both Qi and Blood.

Pathogenesis Analysis: Predominantly due to chronic disease causing the deficiency of Qi and Blood that fails to nourish the tongue body.

2. Stiff Tongue

Characteristics: The tongue has lost its suppleness and flexibility, or is stiff and hard like a board and not able to move freely (Diagram 2-79).

Clinical significance: Primarily seen in the invasion of heat in the Pericardium, or the exhaustion of fluids due to extreme heat, or wind phlegm obstructing the collaterals.

Pathogenesis Analysis: The *Thousand Invaluable Prescriptions • Diseases of the Seven Orifices* points out: "If the tongue is stiff and the patient cannot speak, the disease is in the Organs." which shows that a stiff tongue generally does not indicate a localized pathological change, but is in fact related to the pathological changes of the internal organs. A stiff tongue can also be seen in an externally contracted febrile disease, heat invading the Pericardium and disturbing the Mind, so the tongue lacks control; or the exhaustion of fluids due to extreme heat, the muscles and veins fail to be nourished, hence the tongue body loses its suppleness; or Liver wind with phlegm, wind phlegm obstructing the collaterals, ascending hyperactivity of Liver Yang, muscles and veins lack nourishment, leading to the stiffness of the tongue and its inability to move freely.

A stiff tongue can be subdivided in accordance with the tongue color and the condition of the tongue coating generally as a stiff and deep red tongue with scanty fluids, and a stiff tongue with a thick and greasy coating etc.

2.1   Stiff and Deep Red Tongue with Scanty Fluids

Characteristics: The tongue is stiff and deep red in color and fluid is scanty (Diagram 2-80).

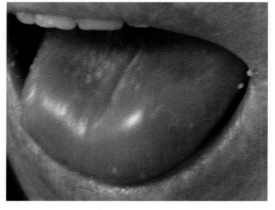

图 2-80 舌色红绛、少津，舌体强硬，舌前部苔剥落（女 脑动脉硬化、脑萎缩）
A deep red tongue with scanty fluids, stiff tongue body, and peeled coating at the anterior of the tongue (female, cerebral artherlosclerosis, encephalatrophy)

【临床意义】 主热盛之证。

【机理分析】 多见于热邪炽盛，伤津耗液，舌体经脉失养。

（二）舌强硬而舌苔厚腻

【舌象特征】 舌体强硬，舌苔厚腻（图2-81）。

【临床意义】 见于风痰阻络，或为中风先兆。

【机理分析】 由于风痰阻络，舌脉失养，则舌体强硬，痰浊上泛于舌面则舌苔厚腻。突然舌强语言謇涩，伴有肢体麻木、眩晕者多为中风先兆。

三、歪斜舌

【舌象特征】 伸舌时舌体偏向一侧，或左或右，称为歪斜舌。一般舌歪在前半部明显（图 2-82，2-83，2-84）。

【临床意义】 多见于中风，中风先兆。

【机理分析】 歪斜舌多由肝风内动，夹痰夹瘀，或痰瘀阻滞一侧舌部经络，而致舌收缩无力，不能伸出，故常见病侧舌肌弛缓，健侧舌肌如常，伸舌时舌体向患侧歪斜。

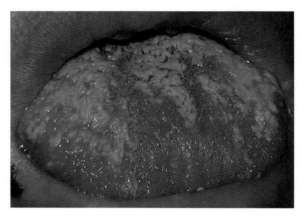

图 2-81　舌红绛，舌体强硬，苔花剥，残留淡黄厚腐苔
（女　脑出血）
A deep red tongue, stiff tongue body, and a patchy peeled coating, the remaining being pale yellow, thick and curdy (female, cerebral hemorrhage)

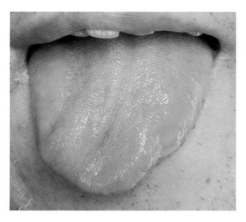

图 2-82　舌色紫暗，舌体歪斜，舌苔淡黄
（男　高血压）
A dull purple and deviated tongue, and a pale yellow tongue coating (male, hypertension)

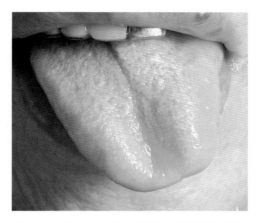

图 2-83　舌色红，舌体歪斜，舌苔薄黄稍腻
（男　脑出血）
A red and deviated tongue, with a thin yellow and slightly greasy tongue coating (male, cerebral hemorrhage)

Clinical significance: Indicating a syndrome of exuberant heat.

Pathogenesis Analysis: Chiefly seen in the exuberance of extreme heat, consuming body fluids, so that the collaterals of the tongue body fail to be nourished.

2. 2   Stiff Tongue with Thick and Greasy Coating

Characteristics: The tongue body is stiff and the tongue coating is thick and greasy (Diagram 2-81).

Clinical significance: Seen in wind phlegm obstructing the collaterals, or a premonitory sign of a wind-stroke.

Pathogenesis Analysis: Due to wind phlegm obstructing the collaterals, the tongue collaterals fail to be nourished, causing the tongue body to become stiff, phlegm turbidity floods upwards to the surface of the tongue leading to a thick and greasy tongue coating. The sudden stiffness of the tongue, difficulty of speech, accompanied by numbness of the body and dizziness are typically the premonitory signs of a wind-stroke.

3. Deviated tongue

Characteristics: A deviated tongue is one that deviates to one side when extended, either to the left or to the right. Generally the deviation is more obvious in the front half of the tongue (Diagram 2-82, 2-83, 2-84).

Clinical significance: Seen in wind stroke or as a premonitory sign of wind stroke.

Pathogenesis Analysis: A deviated tongue is largely due to the internal stirring of Liver wind, interspersed with phlegm and blood stasis, or phlegm and blood stasis obstructing the meridians and collaterals on one side of the tongue, causing weakness of the tongue and its inability to extend or withdraw, thus it is frequently seen that the muscle on one side of the tongue appears lax, and the unaffected side appears normal. The tongue deviates to the affected side on extension.

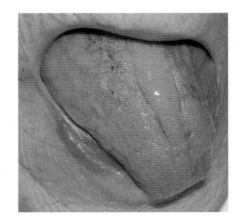

图 2-84   舌色暗红，舌体歪斜，舌苔薄白
（女   脑出血）

A dull red and deviated tongue, and a thin white tongue coating (female, cerebral hemorrhage)

四、颤动舌

【舌象特征】 舌体不自主地震颤抖动，动摇不宁者，称为舌颤动。

【临床意义】 为肝风内动之象。

【机理分析】 风性主动，肝肾阴虚，阴不制阳，肝风内动，或气血亏虚，不能濡养舌体，故见舌体颤动。

五、吐弄舌

【舌象特征】 舌伸于口外，不即回缩者，称为吐舌（图 2-85）。伸舌即回缩，或反复舐口唇四周，掉动不宁者，均称弄舌。

【临床意义】 心脾二经有热。

【机理分析】 心热则动风，脾热则津耗，以致舌吐弄不宁。吐舌可见于疫毒攻心，病情危急时吐舌，多为心气已绝。弄舌多为热盛动风的先兆，吐弄舌也可见于小儿智力发育不全。

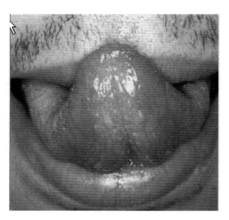

图 2-85 舌色暗红，舌伸于口外不即回缩
（男 高血压、脑梗塞）
A dull red tongue, where on extension of the
tongue it can not be immediately retracted
(male, hypertension, cerebral infarction)

六、短缩舌

【舌象特征】 舌体卷短、紧缩，不能伸长，严重者舌不抵齿者，称为短缩舌。短缩舌常与痿软舌并见（图2-86）。

【临床意义】 多为病情危重的征象。

【机理分析】 舌短缩，色淡白或青紫而湿润，多属寒凝筋脉，或气血虚衰而致舌脉挛缩或舌体失养。总之，短缩舌预示病情危重。

此外，先天性舌系带过短，亦可影响舌体伸出，称为绊舌，无辨证意义。

短缩舌根据舌色、舌形、舌苔情况一般分为舌短缩、色红绛，舌短缩而胖大、苔滑腻。

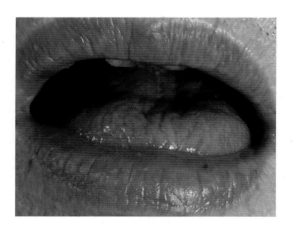

图 2-86 舌色紫红，舌体卷短紧缩不能伸长
（男 中风后遗症）
A purplish red tongue, the tongue body curled, short,
tight and contracted and unable to be extended
(male, sequelae of a stroke)

4. Quivering Tongue

Characteristics: Involuntarily quivering of the tongue without rest is called a quivering tongue.

Clinical significance: It indicates internal stirring of Liver wind.

Pathogenesis Analysis: The nature of wind is to move. Liver and Kidney Yin deficiency, Yin fails to control Yang, and stirs up Liver wind internally, or Qi and Blood deficiency fails to nourish the tongue body, thus the quivering of the tongue.

5. Protruding and Wagging Tongue

Characteristics: The tongue that protrudes out but is unable to retract is called a protruding tongue (Diagram 2-85).

The tongue that protrudes out but immediately withdraws or repeatedly licks the lips or corners of the mouth is called a wagging tongue.

Clinical significance: Heat in the meridians of the Heart and Spleen.

Pathogenesis Analysis: Heart heat stirring up wind and Spleen heat injuring the fluids, causing the protrusion and wagging of the tongue and its inability to be still. A protruding tongue can be seen when a pestilential toxin attacks the Heart. If a protruding tongue is seen when the nature of the disease is critical, this indicates the exhaustion of Heart Qi. A wagging tongue is commonly seen as a premonitory sign of exuberant heat stirring up wind. A protruding and wagging tongue can also be seen in children whose intellect is underdeveloped.

6. Short and Shrunken Tongue

Characteristics: The tongue is contracted, tightened and cannot be fully extended, and in severe cases it cannot even reach the teeth. A short and shrunken tongue is commonly seen together with a flaccid tongue (Diagram 2-86).

Clinical significance: Primarily indicating a critical condition.

Pathogenesis Analysis: A short and shrunken tongue that is pale white or cyanotic in color, and moist is chiefly due to cold obstructing the muscles and veins or due to Qi and Blood deficiency causing the contraction of tongue or failing to nourish the tongue. Overall a short and shrunken tongue is a sign of a critical condition.

Furthermore, there are those who have a congenitally shortened frenulum linguae that can also affect its extension, and these are called stumbling tongues. They have no significance in differential diagnosis.

A short and shrunken tongue can generally be subdivided in accordance with the tongue color, tongue shape and the nature of the tongue coating, namely short shrunken deep red tongue, short shrunken and puffy tongue with a slippery and greasy coating.

（一）舌短缩，色红绛

【舌象特征】 舌体短缩，舌色红绛（图 2-87）。
【临床意义】 热盛伤津。
【机理分析】 多属热盛伤津、筋脉拘急所致。

（二）舌短缩而胖大，苔滑腻

【舌象特征】 舌体短缩而胖大，舌苔滑腻（图 2-88）。
【临床意义】 中风或中风先兆。
【机理分析】 多属痰浊内蕴、风痰阻络。

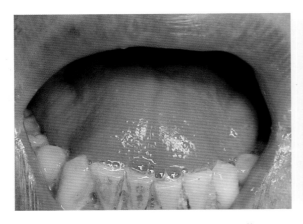 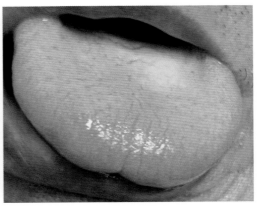

图 2-87　舌色红绛，舌体短缩舌面无苔
（男　结肠癌术后）
A deep red tongue, the tongue body is short
and contracted and coating absent (male,
post-operation for colon cancer)

图 2-88　舌短缩胖大，舌苔白厚腻
（男　脑动脉硬化）
A short tongue and contracted and puffy and
enlarged, with a thick white and greasy coating
(male, cerebral arteriosclerosis)

第五节　舌下络脉

　　舌下络脉是位于舌系带两侧纵行的大络脉，管径一般小于 2.7mm，长度不超过舌下肉阜至舌尖的 3/5，络脉颜色为淡紫色。望舌下络脉主要观察其长度、形态、颜色、粗细、舌下小血络等变化。

　　舌下络脉的观察方法是：先让病人张口，将舌体向上腭方向翘起，舌尖可轻抵上腭，勿用力太过，使舌体保持自然松弛，舌下络脉充分显露。首先观察舌系带两侧的大络脉粗细、颜色，有否怒张、弯曲等改变。然后再查看周围细小络脉的颜色、形态以及有无紫暗的珠状结节。

6. 1 Short and Shrunken, Deep Red Tongue

Characteristics: The tongue body is short and shrunken, deep red in color (Diagram 2-87).

Clinical significance: Indicating the exuberance heat consuming body fluids.

Pathogenesis Analysis: Predominantly due to exuberance heat consuming fluids, and contraction of the muscles.

6. 2 Short, Shrunken and Puffy Tongue with Slippery and Greasy Coating

Characteristics: The tongue is short and shrunken yet puffy, and the tongue coating is slippery and greasy(Diagram 2-88).

Clinical significance: Indicating wind-stroke or the premonitory sign of a wind-stroke.

Pathogenesis Analysis: Predominantly due to the accumulation of turbid phlegm, and wind phlegm obstructing the collaterals.

SECTION FIVE   VESSELS UNDER THE TONGUE (SUBLINGUAL VEINS)

The vessels under the tongue are located on both sides and parallel to the frenulum linguae. These are the large vessels, pale purple in color, whose diameter is generally no bigger than 2. 7mm, whose length is no longer than 3/5 of the length starting from the sublingual papillae to the tip of the tongue. Inspection of the vessels below the tongue mainly includes changes of the length, shape, color, thickness and the smaller vessels under the tongue etc.

The method for inspection of the vessels is: for the patient to have their mouth open, the tongue curled upwards towards the palate with the tip of the tongue gently resting on the palate, done without excessive force so that the tongue body can retain its natural slack, so that the vessels are suitably visible. Firstly inspect for changes of the large vessels beside the frenulum in the thickness, color, curvature, or whether they are swollen etc. Thereafter, the color and form of the smaller vessels surrounding the large vessels should be inspected with the observation of whether the dark purple bead-like protuberances occur.

　　舌下络脉异常及其临床意义：舌下络脉细而短，色淡红，周围小络脉不明显，舌色和舌下黏膜色偏淡者，多属气血不足（图2-89）。

　　舌下络脉粗胀，或舌下络脉呈青紫、紫红、绛紫、紫黑色，或舌下细小络脉呈暗红色或紫色网状，或舌下络脉曲张如紫色珠子大小不等的瘀血结节等改变，都是血瘀的征象。其形成原因可有寒、热、气滞、痰湿、阳虚等不同，需进一步结合其他症状进行分析（图2-90，2-91，2-92）。

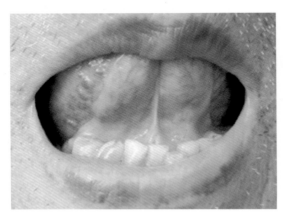

图 2-89　舌下络脉细而短，色淡

（男　高血压病）

The vessels under the tongue are small and short,
and pale in color（male，hypertension）

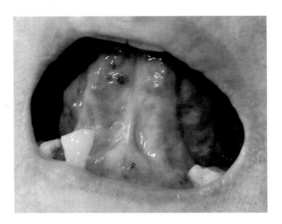

图 2-90　舌下络脉曲张，色紫黑

（女　脑动脉硬化，脑萎缩）

The vessels under the tongue are enlarged,
and purplish-black in color（female，cerebral
arteriosclerosis，encephalatrophy）

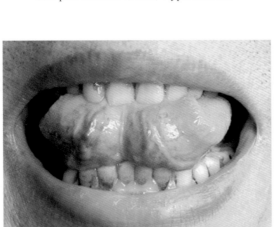

图 2-91　舌下络脉瘀紫曲张

（男　高血压病）

The vessels under the tongue are bruise-like
purple in color and enlarged（male，hypertension）

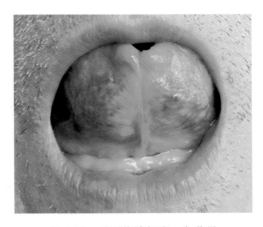

图 2-92　舌下络脉粗胀，色紫黑

（男　脑动脉硬化）

The vessels under the tongue are thickened,
and purplish-black in color（male，cerebral
arteriosclerosis）

The abnormality of the sublingual veins and their clinical significance: If the vessels are thin and short, pale red in color, and the surrounding smaller vessels are not distinct, the tongue color and the mucous membrane underneath the tongue both tend to be pale, this generally indicates the deficiency of Qi and Blood (Diagram 2-89).

If the vessels are thick, cyanotic, or purplish red, or purplish dark red, or purplish black in color, or the smaller vessels are a dull red or purple in color and meshed like a net, or the enlargement of the vessels under the tongue with small bead like purple protuberances on the vessels that vary in size, all lead to the stasis of Blood. The cause of these formations is cold, heat, Qi stagnation, phlegm dampness, Yang deficiency etc. Thus it is necessary to take one step further by analyzing in conjunction with other signs and symptoms (Diagram 2-90, 2-91, 2-92).

第三章

望 舌 苔

舌苔，指舌面上的一层苔状物，舌苔是脾胃之气上蒸胃阴而成。正常的舌苔，应该是薄白均匀、干湿适中。病理性的舌苔多由胃中腐浊之气上泛而成。由于人的胃气有强弱不同、感邪有寒热之分，故可形成各种不同的病理性舌苔。望舌苔要注意苔质和苔色两方面的变化。

第一节 苔 质

苔质即舌苔的质地、形态。主要观察舌苔的厚薄、润燥、腻腐、剥落、偏全、真假等方面的改变。

一、薄、厚苔

舌苔的厚薄是以"见底"、"不见底"作为衡量标准。薄、厚苔主要反映邪正的盛衰和病位的浅深。

（一）薄苔

【舌象特征】 透过舌苔能隐隐见到舌体的苔称为薄苔，又称见底苔（图 3-1，3-2，3-3）。

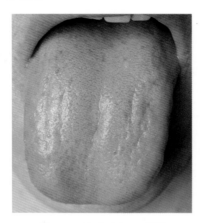

图 3-1 舌色暗红，苔薄
（女 冠状动脉粥样硬化性心脏病）
A dull red tongue, and a thin coating (female, coronary artherosclerotic heart disease)

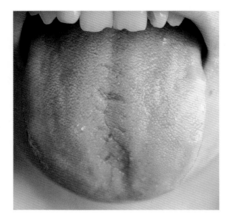

图 3-2 舌色淡红，舌面前部有浅裂纹，苔薄白
（女 冠状动脉粥样硬化性心脏病）
A pale red tongue, with shallow fissures on the anterior of the tongue, and a thin white coating (female, coronary artherosclerotic heart disease)

CHAPTER THREE

INSPECTING THE TONGUE COATING

Tongue coating refers to the layer of moss-like substance covering the surface of the tongue. It is the by-product from the fumigation of Stomach Yin from the Spleen and Stomach. The normal tongue coating should be thin, white, evenly distributed, and slightly moist, that isn't too dry or too damp. The pathological nature of the tongue coating is mainly due to the Qi of the Stomach's excessive turbidity arising to form on the tongue. Due to differences in strength of each individual's Stomach Qi, and the different natures of heat and cold pathogens, this will result in the variation of the formation of pathological tongue coatings. The inspection of the tongue coating should encompass changes in its nature and color.

SECTION ONE   TONGUE COATING PROPER

The tongue coating proper refers to its texture and form. Examination of the tongue coating mainly includes changes in its thickness, moisture, greasiness and curdy (moldiness), peeling, distribution whether it is uniform or partial, and whether it is a true or false coating.

1. Thin, Thick Coating

The standard for measuring the thickness of a tongue coating is whether it is "base visible" or "base invisible".

Generally speaking, the degree of thickness of a tongue coating reflects on the strength or weakness of the anti-pathogenic Qi and pathogenic factor, and also the depth in which the disease is located.

1.1   Thin Coating

Characteristics: A thin coating, also named base visible tongue is one in which the tongue body is faintly visible through the coating itself (Diagram 3-1, 3-2, 3-3).

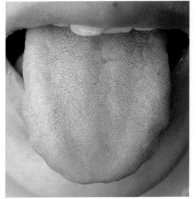

图 3-3 舌色红，苔薄
（女 糖尿病）
A red tongue, and a thin coating
(female, diabetes)

【临床意义】 主外感表证、内伤轻证。

【机理分析】 薄苔见于正常人，多提示胃有生发之气；疾病过程中见之也多说明邪气不盛，主表证、轻证。

（二）厚苔

【舌象特征】 不能透过舌苔见到舌质之苔称为厚苔，又称不见底苔（图3-4，3-5）。

【临床意义】 邪盛入里，或内有痰湿、食积、里热等证。

【机理分析】 厚苔是由胃气夹湿浊、痰湿、食滞等邪气熏蒸所致。《辨舌指南·辨舌之苔垢》说："苔垢薄者，形气不足；苔垢厚者，病气有余。"

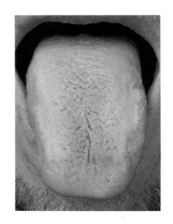 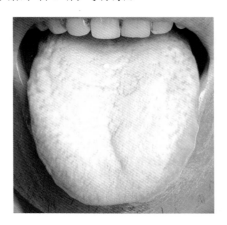

图3-4 舌色暗红，舌苔黄厚腐　　　　　　　图3-5 舌苔淡黄厚腐
（男　慢性肝炎）　　　　　　　　　　　　（男　右颞硬膜血块）

A dull red tongue, and a thick yellow and　　A thick, pale yellow and curdy tongue coating
curdy coating (male, chronic hepatitis)　　　　（male, right temporal intradural clot）

辨舌苔厚薄可测邪气的盛衰。《辨舌指南·辨舌之苔垢》曰："苔薄者，表邪初见；苔厚者，里滞已深。"疾病初起在表，病情轻浅，未伤胃气，舌苔亦无明显变化，可见到薄苔；或内伤病较轻，胃气未伤，舌苔没有明显变化，也可见之。舌苔厚或舌中根部尤著者，多提示外感病邪已入里，或胃肠内有宿食、痰浊停滞，主病位在里，病情较重。

辨舌苔厚薄可测病位的深浅。舌苔由薄变厚，提示邪气渐盛，为病进，病位由浅入深；舌苔由厚渐化，舌上复生薄白新苔，提示正气胜邪，为病退，病位由深入浅。

舌苔的厚薄转化，一般是渐变的过程，如薄苔突然增厚，提示邪气极盛，迅速入里；厚苔骤然消退，舌上无新生薄苔，为正不胜邪，或胃气暴绝。

二、润、燥苔

舌苔润燥主要反映体内津液盈亏和输布情况。主要有润苔、滑苔、燥苔、糙苔4种。

Clinical significance: Indicating an externally contracted superficial syndrome, or a mild internal impairment syndrome.

Pathogenesis Analysis: A thin coating seen in a healthy individual suggests that the Qi of the Stomach is functioning normally. If seen during the course of a disease, it suggests that the pathogenic factor is weak, indicating an external and mild syndrome.

1.2   Thick Coating

Characteristics: A thick coating also named base invisible tongue is one in which the tongue proper is not visible through the coating, (Diagram 3-4,3-5).

Clinical significance: Indicating the exuberance and internal invasion of the pathogenic factors, or the internal stagnation of phlegm and dampness, food stagnation, or internal heat syndrome etc.

Pathogenesis Analysis: A thick coating is due to the fermentation of Stomach Qi interspersed with pathogenic factors such as turbid damp, phlegm damp, food stagnation etc. *Guide to Tongue Differentiation • Differentiating turbid Coatings of the Tongue* states: "If the tongue coating is dirty and thin, it means that the body's Qi is weak. If it is dirty and thick, it means that the pathogenic factor is strong."

Differentiating the thickness of tongue coating can give an indication of the strength of the pathogenic factor. *Guide to Tongue Differentiation • Differentiating turbid Coatings of the Tongue* states: "If the coating is thin, the pathogenic factor is just beginning to manifest; if the coating is thick, the pathogenic factor is deep inside." During the initial stages of a disease in the exterior, the nature of the disease is mild and superficial, not yet to injure Stomach Qi, there is no obvious change to the tongue coating, thus a thin coating is seen; or it can also be seen in an internal impairment disease that is comparatively mild where the Stomach Qi has not yet to be injured, thus no significant change to the tongue coating. A thick tongue coating or coating that is thicker on the centre and root of the tongue indicates the exogenous pathogenic factor has invaded the interior, or there is food stagnation in the Stomach and Intestines, stagnation of turbid phlegm, signifying that the location of the disease is in the interior and the disease is relatively severe.

Differentiating the thickness of tongue coating can give an indication of the depth in which the disease is located. If the tongue coating changes from thin to thick, it indicates that the pathogenic factor is gradually getting stronger, the disease is progressing, the disease is transferring from the exterior to the interior. If the tongue coating gradually changes from thick to a thin, white and new coating, it indicates that the anti-pathogenic Qi is defeating the pathogenic factor, the disease is receding, and the disease is moving from the interior to the exterior.

Generally, the transformation of a thick coating or thin coating is a gradual process. If a thin coating suddenly changes to a thick coating, it indicates the extreme exuberance of the pathogenic factor and its rapid penetration into the interior. If a coating suddenly changes from thick to thin and the tongue has no new, thin coating, this indicates that the anti-pathogenic Qi cannot defeat the pathogenic factor, or the sudden collapse of Stomach Qi.

2. Moist, Dry Coating

The moisture of the tongue coating primarily reflects on the condition of body fluids, of its abundance, decline, and distribution in the body. There are mainly 4 types, a moist coating, slippery coating, dry coating, and rough coating.

（一）润苔

【舌象特征】 舌苔干湿适中，不滑不燥，称为润苔（图3-6，3-7）。

【临床意义】 是正常舌苔的表现之一，疾病过程中见之，反映体内津液未伤。

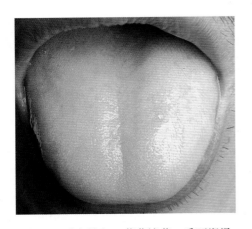

图 3-6　舌色淡红，苔薄淡黄，舌面润泽
（男　慢性粒细胞白血病）

A light red tongue, with a thin pale yellow
coating, and a moist tongue surface
(male, chronic granulocytic leukemia)

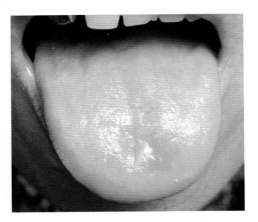

图 3-7　舌色淡红，舌面润
（男　脑梗塞、高血压）

A light red tongue, with a moist tongue surface
(male, cerebral infarction, hypertension)

【机理分析】 润苔是正常舌苔的表现之一，为胃津、肾液上承，布露舌面的表现。若疾病过程中见到润苔，提示体内津液未伤，如风寒表证、湿证初起、食滞、瘀血等均可见润苔。

（二）滑苔

【舌象特征】 舌面水分过多，伸舌欲滴，扪之湿而滑，称为滑苔（图3-8，3-9，3-10）。

【临床意义】 主寒、主湿、主痰饮。

【机理分析】 滑苔为水湿之邪内聚的表现，主寒、主湿、主痰饮。如脾阳不振，寒湿内生，湿聚为痰饮，随经脉上溢于舌苔，故可出现滑苔。

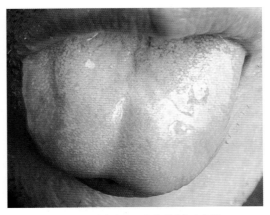

图 3-8　舌色红，舌苔黄腻而水滑
（男　冠状动脉粥样硬化性心脏病、房颤）

A red tongue, and a greasy yellow and watery
and slippery tongue coating (male, coronary
artherosclerotic heart disease, atrial fibrillation)

2.1   Moist Coating

Characteristics: A moist coating is one that is adequately moist, that isn't too damp or too dry (Diagram 3-6,3-7).

Clinical significance: A moist tongue coating is one of the manifestations of a normal tongue. If seen during the course of a disease, it indicates that the body fluids have not yet to be consumed.

Pathogenesis Analysis: A moist coating is seen in a normal tongue, being the transportation and distribution of the Stomach and Kidney fluids up to the surface of the tongue. If a moist tongue coating is seen during the course of a disease, it indicates that the body fluids are not impaired. For instance, an exogenous wind cold syndrome, the initial stages of a damp syndrome, food stagnation, blood stasis etc. can all present with a moist tongue coating.

2.2   Slippery Coating

Characteristics: A slippery coating is excessively wet, and dribbles on extension of the tongue. If the tongue coating should be felt, it would feel wet and slippery (Diagram 3-8, 3-9,3-10).

Clinical significance: Indicates cold, damp, or phlegm fluid retention.

Pathogenesis Analysis: A slippery coating is the manifestation of internal accumulation of dampness, indicating cold, damp, or phlegm fluid retention. The depression of Spleen Yang leads to the internal production of damp cold, accumulation of damp leading to the retention of phlegm fluid that trails the meridians to flood up to the tongue coating, thus presenting a slippery coating.

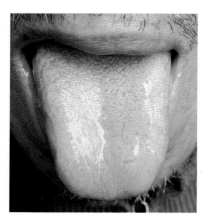

图 3-9   舌色暗红，舌苔淡黄，舌面水滑
（男   冠状动脉粥样硬化性心脏病、房颤）
A dull red tongue, with a pale yellow tongue coating, and a watery and slippery tongue surface (male, coronary artherosclerotic heart disease, atrial fibrillation)

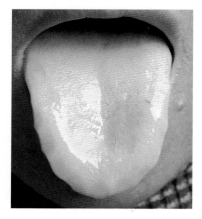

图 3-10   舌色淡红，舌面水滑，苔根薄黄
（女   慢性肾功能不全）
A light red tongue, a watery and slippery tongue surface, and a thin yellow coating at the root (female, chronic renal insufficiency)

（三）燥苔

【舌象特征】 舌苔干燥，扪之无津，甚则舌苔干裂，称为燥苔（图 3-11）。

【临床意义】 高热、大汗、吐泻、痰饮瘀血内阻等。

【机理分析】 燥苔提示体内津液已伤。如高热、大汗、吐泻后，或过服温燥药物等，导致津液不足，舌苔失于滋润而干燥。亦有因阳气为阴邪（痰饮水湿等）所阻，不能上蒸津液濡润舌苔而见燥苔者，是津液失于输布之象。因此，燥苔主病多见热盛伤津、阳虚气不化津。

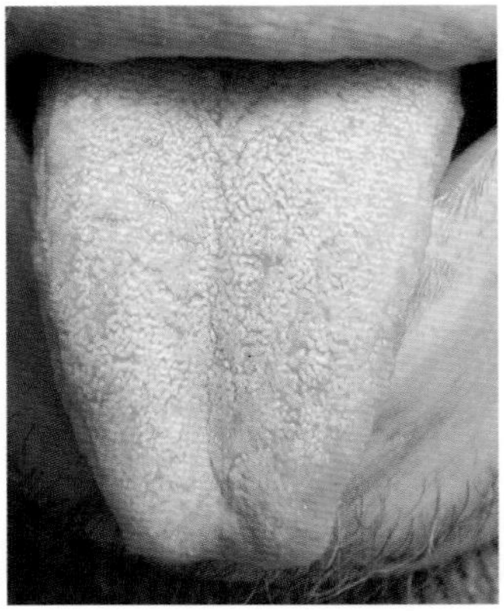

（四）糙苔

【舌象特征】 苔质粗糙，扪之碍手，称为糙苔（图 3-12，3-13）。

【临床意义】 见于热盛伤津之重症；或为秽浊之邪盘踞中焦。

【机理分析】 糙苔可由燥苔进一步发展而成。舌苔干结粗糙，津液全无，多见于热盛伤津、舌面失养之重症；苔质粗糙而不干者，多为秽浊之邪盘踞中焦。

图 3-11 舌色红，舌苔淡黄而燥
（男 急性肾小球肾炎）
A red tongue, and a pale yellow and dry tongue coating (male, acute glomenular nephritis)

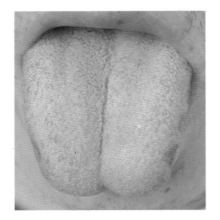

图 3-12 舌色红，苔薄白而糙
（男 肾病综合征）
A red tongue, and a thin white and rough coating (male, nephrotic syndrome)

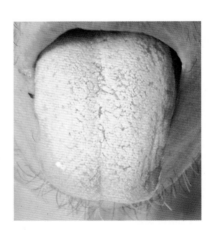

图 3-13 舌色红，苔白带黄糙
（男 胆囊炎）
A red tongue, and a white yellow and rough coating (male, cholecystitis)

2. 3   Dry Coating

Characteristics: A dry coating has insufficient fluids. If the coating is palpated, it will feel dry and in severe cases it can be dry and cracked (Diagram 3-11).

Clinical significance: Indicating exuberant heat, profuse sweating, vomiting and diarrhea, internal obstruction of phlegm rheum, blood stasis, etc.

Pathogenesis Analysis: A dry coating signifies the consumption of body fluids. If there is exuberant heat, or following profuse sweating, vomiting, diarrhea, or excessive consumption of warm and dry natured medication etc. leading to the deficiency of body fluids, the tongue coating loses nourishment and moistening and becomes dry. It can also be due to the obstruction of Yang Qi by Yin pathogenic factors (phlegm, fluid, dampness etc.). The Yang Qi is then unable to transform and transport the fluids upwards to the tongue failing to moisten the tongue coating and as a result the coating becomes dry. This is a manifestation of the failure to distribute body fluids. Therefore a dry coating generally indicates a disease with exuberant heat and the consumption of body fluids, or Yang deficiency failing to transform the body fluids.

2. 4   Rough Coating

Characteristics: A rough coating is rough and coarse, and when touched, it feels unsmooth (Diagram 3-12,3-13).

Clinical significance: Seen in a severe syndrome of exuberant heat and consumption of body fluids or the stagnation of filthy turbidity in the middle energizer.

Pathogenesis Analysis: A rough coating can be the result of the progression of a dry coating. A dry and rough tongue coating and completely absence of fluids is seen in a severe syndrome of exuberant heat and consumption of body fluids. A rough coating that is not dry is seen in the stagnation of filthy turbidity in the middle energizer.

三、腐、腻苔

腐、腻苔是舌苔质地改变的表现之一，根据苔的质地及颜色一般分为腐苔、腻苔两种。

（一）腐苔

【舌象特征】 苔质颗粒疏松、粗大而厚，如豆腐渣堆铺舌面，揩之可去，称为腐苔（图 3-14，3-15，3-16，3-17）。

【临床意义】 主食积胃肠，或痰浊内蕴。

【机理分析】 腐苔的形成，多因邪热有余，蒸腾胃中腐浊之气上泛，聚集于舌，主食积胃肠，或痰浊内蕴。

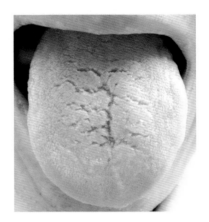

图 3-14　舌色淡红，舌苔灰厚而腐，苔深裂（男　2 型糖尿病）
A light red tongue, with a thick gray and curdy coating, and deep fissures on the coating (male, type Ⅱ diabetes)

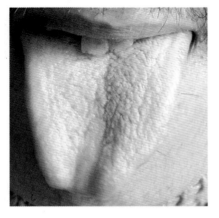

图 3-15　舌色淡红，舌苔淡黄腐而厚（男　慢性胃炎）
A light red tongue, and a thick pale yellow and curdy tongue coating (male, chronic gastritis)

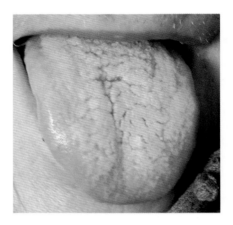

图 3-16　舌色紫暗，舌苔黄厚腐浊（男　肺源性心脏病）
A dull purple tongue, and a thick yellow, curdy and turbid tongue coating (male, corpulmonale)

3. Curdy and Greasy Coating

A greasy or curdy coating is one of the manifestations of changes in the tongue coating proper. They are categorized in accordance with the coating proper and color generally into 2 types: curdy coating, and greasy coating.

3.1 Curdy Coating

Characteristics: The tongue coating proper is composed of thick, coarse granules loosely scattered like a layer of bean curd dregs, which can be easily scraped off is called curdy and moldy coating (Diagram 3-14,3-15,3-16,3-17).

Clinical significance: Indicating food stagnation in the Stomach and Intestines, or the internal accumulation of turbid phlegm.

Pathogenesis Analysis: The formation of a curdy coating is predominantly due to excess pathogenic heat fumigating the turbid and curdy Stomach Qi upwards to accumulate on the tongue, accumula-

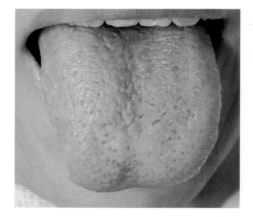

图 3-17 舌色红，舌尖有红点，苔灰黄厚腐腻
（女 肺癌伴脑转移）
A red tongue, with red spots on the tongue tip, and
a thick grayish yellow, curdy and greasy coating
(female, lung cancer metastasized to the brain)

tion of food in the Stomach and intestine, or the internal accumulation of phlegm turbidity.

（二）腻苔

【舌象特征】 苔质颗粒细小、质地致密、紧贴舌面，揩之不去，刮之不易脱落者，称为腻苔（图 3-18，3-19，3-20，3-21，3-22）。

【临床意义】 主湿浊、痰饮、食积。

【机理分析】 腻苔多由湿浊内蕴、阳气被遏、湿浊上泛舌面所致。

腻苔还可根据苔色不同而分为以下几种：

1. 白腻而滑苔

【舌象特征】 舌苔白腻而滑（图 3-23）。

【临床意义】 主痰浊、寒湿。

【机理分析】 舌苔白腻而滑者，为痰浊、寒湿内阻，阳气被遏，气机阻滞。

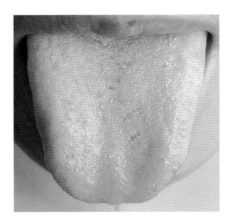

图 3-18　舌色淡红，舌苔色白而细腻
（女　淋巴瘤）
A light red tongue, and a white and slightly greasy tongue coating (female, lymphoma)

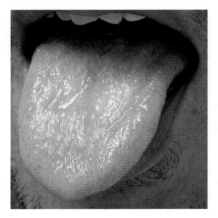

图 3-19　舌色红，舌尖有芒刺，苔黄厚腻
（男　脑血管意外后遗症）
A red tongue, with prickles on the tongue tip, and a thick yellow and greasy coating (male, sequelae of a cerebrovascular trauma)

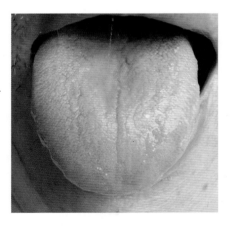

图 3-20　舌色淡红，舌苔深黄腻
（男　食管癌）
A light red tongue, and a greasy deep yellow tongue coating (male, esophageal cancer)

3.2 Greasy Coating

Characteristics：A greasy coating proper is composed of small and compact granules on the surface of the tongue that are difficult to scrape off or exfoliate (Diagram 3-18, 3-19, 3-20, 3-21, 3-22).

Clinical significance：Indicates turbid dampness, phlegm fluid retention, and food stagnation.

Pathogenesis Analysis：Chiefly due to accumulation of turbid dampness obstructing Yang Qi, and turbid phlegm rising upwards to the surface of the tongue.

Greasy coating can also be categorized according to the color of the coating as the following.

3.2.1 Greasy White and Slippery Coating

Characteristics：The tongue coating is white, greasy and slippery (Diagram 3-23).

Clinical significance：It suggests turbid phlegm, damp cold.

Pathogenesis Analysis：Due to the stagnation of turbid phlegm,

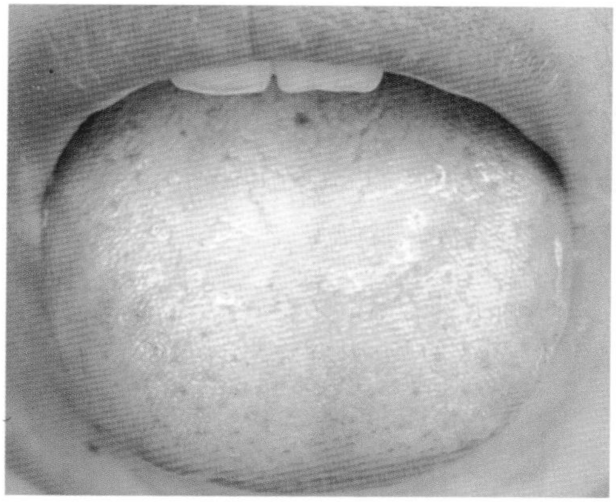

图 3-21 舌色红，舌苔中部淡黄厚腻
（女 慢性肾小球肾炎）
A red tongue, and a thick pale yellow and greasy tongue coating in the centre (female, chronic glomerular nephritis)

and damp cold causing the obstruction of Yang Qi, and obstruction of Qi-activity.

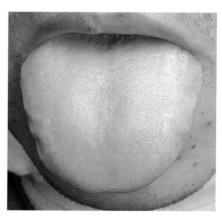

图 3-22 舌色淡红，舌苔淡黄细腻
（男 高血压病）
A light red tongue, and a pale yellow and slightly greasy tongue coating (male, hypertension)

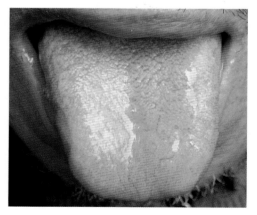

图 3-23 舌色暗红，舌苔白腻水滑
（男 乏力待查）
A dull red tongue, and a greasy white, watery and slippery tongue coating (male, lassitude awaiting examination)

2．白厚黏腻苔

【舌象特征】 舌苔白厚黏腻（图 3-24）。

【临床意义】 主湿邪、痰浊内蕴。

【机理分析】 舌苔厚而黏腻者，是脾胃湿浊内蕴、邪气上泛所致。

3．黄腻而厚苔

【舌象特征】 舌苔黄腻而厚（图 3-25）。

【临床意义】 湿热、痰热、暑湿等。

【机理分析】 当痰湿浊邪化热时，还可在苔色上反映出，如舌苔黄腻而厚，为湿热、痰热、暑湿等邪内蕴，熏蒸上泛于舌。

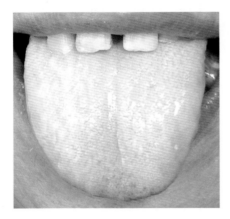

图 3-24　舌色淡红，舌尖芒刺，苔白厚黏腻
（男　慢性肾小球肾炎）

A light red tongue, prickles on the tongue tip,
and a thick white, sticky and greasy coating
(male, chronic glomerular nephritis)

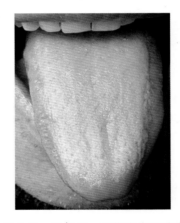

图 3-25　舌质红，舌苔淡黄而厚腻
（男　急性胃炎）

A red tongue proper, and a thick pale yellow
and greasy tongue coating (male, acute gastritis)

四、剥苔

【舌象特征】 舌苔全部或部分剥落，剥落处舌面光滑无苔者，称为剥苔。剥苔根据剥落的部位、程度、范围一般分为前剥苔、中剥苔、根剥苔、花剥苔、镜面舌、类剥苔、地图舌 7 种情况。与舌色相关的有镜面舌红舌、镜面舌淡舌。

舌前部苔剥落者，称前剥苔（图 3-26）；舌中苔剥落者，称中剥苔（图 3-27，3-28，3-29）；舌根部苔剥者，称根剥苔（图 3-30）；舌苔多处剥落，舌面仅斑驳片存少量舌苔者，称花剥苔（图 3-31）；舌苔全部剥落，舌面光滑如镜者，称为镜面舌，是剥苔最严重的一种（图 3-32，3-33）；舌苔剥落处，舌面不光滑，仍有新生苔质颗粒或乳头可见者，称类剥苔（图 3-34）。舌苔大片剥落，边缘突起，界限清楚，剥落部位时时转移，称为地图舌（图 3-35，3-36）。

【临床意义】 一般主胃气匮乏，胃阴枯涸或气血两虚。

3.2.2 Thick White Greasy Coating

Characteristics: Tongue coating is thick, white and greasy (Diagram 3-24).

Clinical significance: Indicates pathogenic factor dampness, internal stagnation of turbid phlegm.

Pathogenesis Analysis: A thick white and greasy coating suggests stagnation of turbid dampness in the Spleen and Stomach spreading upwards to the tongue.

3.2.3 Thick Yellow and Greasy Coating

Characteristics: Tongue coating is yellow, greasy, and thick (Diagram 3-25).

Clinical significance: Indicates damp heat, phlegm heat, or summer damp.

Pathogenesis Analysis: When the pathogenic turbid phlegm damp transforms heat it can be reflected on the coating and its color. Thus thick, yellow, and greasy coating is the accumulation of damp heat, phlegm heat or summer dampness etc. internal accumulation of pathogenic factors, steaming upwards to the tongue.

4. Peeled Coating

Characteristics: Tongue coating that is completely or partially peeled, is called a peeled tongue coating. At the site of the peeled coating the surface of tongue appears shiny and slippery. Due to the different regions of the peeled coating and the different sizes, the types of peeled tongue coatings are divided into 7 types: peeled anterior coating, peeled center coating, peeled root coating, patchy peeled coating, minor-like tongue, peeled-like coating, mapped tongue. Concerning tongue color is a minor-like and red tongue, and a mirror-like and pale tongue.

The anterior part of the coating is peeled, which is named peeled anterior coating (Diagram 3-26). If the center of the coating is peeled, it is named peeled center coating (Diagram 3-27, 3-28, 3-29). If the root of the coating is peeled, it is named peeled root coating (Diagram 3-30). If the regions of peeled coating are scattered, and the surface of the tongue is mottled with only a small amount of tongue coating, it is named patchy peeled coating (Diagram 3-31).

If the tongue coating is completely peeled, the tongue surface appears shiny and slippery. It is one of the most severe types of peeled coatings with the name of Mirror-Like Tongue (Diagram 3-32, 3-33).

The areas of the tongue surface where coating is peeled are not shiny and slippery, with a granule of new coating or papillae. It is named peeled-like coating (Diagram 3-34).

Where a big piece of coating is peeled, the borders of the peeled coating protrude are clear, and the area of the peeled coating changes constantly. It is named mapped tongue (Diagram 3-35, 3-36).

Clinical Significance: It is generally an indication of Stomach Qi deficiency, exhaustion of Stomach Yin or the deficiency of Qi and Blood.

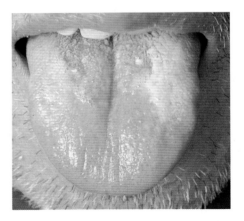

图 3-26 舌红，苔中前剥，苔色淡黄腐腻
（男 多发性骨髓瘤）

A red tongue, with a coating that is peeled at
the centre and anterior, and that is pale yellow,
curdy and greasy (male, multiple myeloma)

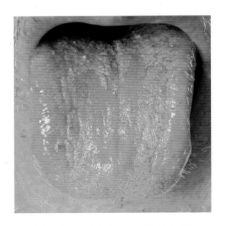

图 3-27 舌色红，舌苔前中剥
（男 再生障碍性贫血）

A red tongue, with a tongue coating
that is peeled at the centre and anterior
(male, aplastic anemia)

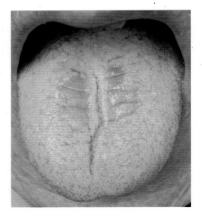

图 3-28 舌色暗红，舌苔淡黄腻，中花剥
（男 慢性胃炎）

A dull red tongue, with a greasy pale yellow
tongue coating that is patchy and peeled
at the centre (male, chronic gastritis)

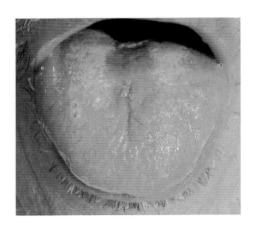

图 3-29 舌色紫，苔前中剥
（男 急性非淋巴细胞性白血病）

A purple tongue, with a coating that is
peeled at the anterior and centre (male,
acute non-lymphocytic leukemia)

【机理分析】 剥落苔的形成，总因胃气阴两虚，不能上蒸于舌面所致。鉴于胃气、胃阴损伤的程度不同，因而形成各种不同形状的剥落苔。

五、偏全苔

根据舌苔在舌面的分布情况分为全苔、偏苔两种。

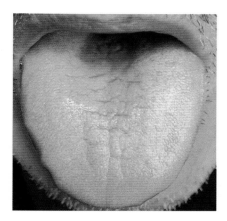

图 3-30　舌色红，苔黄根剥
（男　慢性支气管炎急性发作）

A red tongue, with a yellow coating that is peeled at
the root (male, acute attack of chronic bronchitis)

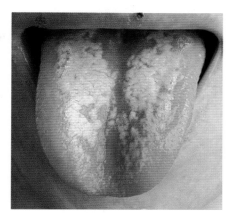

图 3-31　舌色鲜红，苔淡黄而花剥
（女　慢性胃肠炎）

A bright red tongue, with a pale yellow and patchy
peeled coating (female, chronic gastroenteritis)

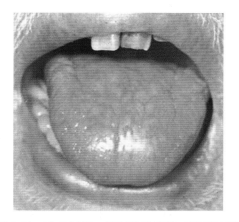

图 3-32　舌色红绛，舌面光剥无苔（镜面红舌）
（男　肺癌）

A deep red tongue, with a shiny tongue surface
where the coating is completely peeled and absent
(a mirror-like red tongue)(male, lung cancer)

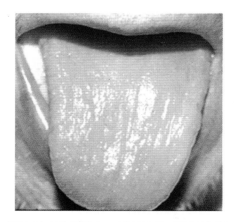

图 3-33　舌色淡白，舌面无苔（镜面淡舌）
（男　淋巴瘤）

A pale white tongue, and an absence of coating
(A mirror-like pale tongue) (male, lymphoma)

Pathogenesis Analysis：The formation of a peeled coating is primarily due to the deficiency of Qi and Yin of the Stomach that fails to vaporize upwards to the tongue surface. Due to the difference in severity and degree of the impairment of Qi and Yin of the Stomach, thus the different types of peeled coating are formated.

5. Complete or Partial Coating

A complete or partial coating is categorized according to the condition of the distribution of the coating on the tongue surface as complete coating, or partial coating.

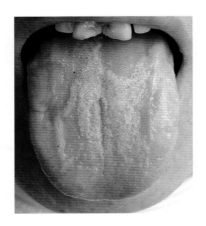

图 3-34　舌色淡红，舌苔白，舌苔剥落处可见
新生颗粒（类剥苔）（男　萎缩性胃炎）
A light red tongue, with a white tongue coating,
and granules of new coating can be seen in the areas
where the coating is peeled（peeled coating type）
（male, atrophic gastritis）

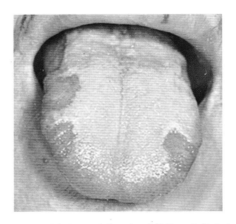

图 3-35　舌色红，舌苔不规则脱落，边缘突起，
苔色淡黄（地图舌）（慢性胃炎）
A red tongue, with a peeled tongue coating that is
irregular with prominent edges; and the coating is
pale yellow（mapped tongue）（chronic gastritis）

（一）全苔

【舌象特征】　舌苔满布舌面，称为全苔
（图 3-37，3-38）。

【临床意义】　诊邪之盛衰。

【机理分析】　病中见全苔，常主邪气弥
漫，多为湿邪、痰浊内阻。

（二）偏苔

【舌象特征】　舌苔仅布于舌的前、后、
左、右之某一局部称为偏苔（图 3-39）。

【临床意义】　察舌苔分布偏在何部，可
诊病变之所在。

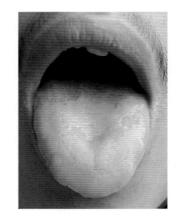

图 3-36　舌色淡红，质嫩，舌苔剥落，
边缘突起，苔色淡白（男　乏力待查）
A light red and tender tongue, with a pale
white coating that is peeled with prominent
edges（male, lassitude awaiting examination）

【机理分析】　偏外苔（舌尖为外），是邪
气入里未深，而胃气先伤；偏内苔（舌根属
内），是表邪虽减，胃滞依然；若仅见中根部有苔，为痰饮、食滞停留中焦；舌苔偏
于左右一侧，为邪在半表半里，或为肝胆湿热。

若因咀嚼习惯而苔偏于一侧，或因牙齿脱落而使一侧舌苔偏厚，与病理性偏苔
要作区别。偏苔与剥落苔也不同，偏苔为舌苔分布上的病理现象，而剥落苔是因病
而致某一部位舌苔剥落，使舌苔显示偏于某处。

5.1 Complete Coating

Characteristics: The tongue coating is evenly and completely distributed over the surface of the tongue (Diagram 3-37, 3-38).

Clinical significance: To determine the strength of a pathogenic factor during pathological changes.

Pathogenesis Analysis: If seen during the course of a disease, it generally indicates that the pathogenic factor is spread all over, chiefly due to damp pathogen, internal stagnation of turbid phlegm.

5.2 Partial Coating

Characteristics: The tongue coating is distributed only over the front, back, left, right, or any one part of the tongue (Diagram 3-39).

Clinical significance: Observing the area in which there is tongue coating can determine the location of the pathological change.

Pathogenesis Analysis: Outer (being the tip of the tongue) coating indicates that although the pathogenic factor has invaded the interior it is still not too deep, and Stomach Qi is the first to be injured; an inner (being the root of the tongue) coating indicates that although the superficial pathogenic factor has receded, stagnation in the Stomach is still present; if coating is seen only on the centre and root of the tongue, this indicates retention of phlegm fluid, or food stagnation in the middle energizer; if the tongue coating is on one side of the tongue, either left or right, this indicates that the pathogenic factor is in the half exterior and half interior level, or being damp heat of the Liver and Gall Bladder.

Chewing habits, or fragmented teeth can

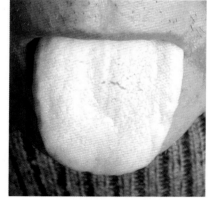

图 3-37 舌苔白厚腻，满布舌面
（男 肺炎球菌肺炎）

A tongue coating that is thick, white and greasy, and distributed completely over the tongue surface
(male, pneumococcal pneumonia)

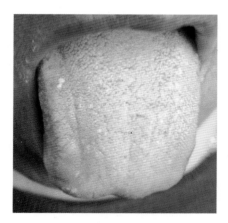

图 3-38 舌色红，舌苔满布舌面
（女 腹痛待查）

A red tongue, and a tongue coating that is distributed completely over the tongue surface
(female, abdominal pain awaiting examination)

also cause partial tongue coating to be thicker on the side of the tongue, thus it is important to differentiate this with a pathological partial tongue coating. A partial coating is different from a peeled coating, a partial coating is tongue coating that has been distributed as the pathological manifestation, while a peeled coating is caused by disease leading to the coating to be peeled in certain areas, making it appear as if the tongue coating is partial to certain areas.

六、真假苔

判断舌苔的真假，以有根无根为标准。一般分为真苔、假苔两种。

（一）真苔

【舌象特征】 舌苔紧贴舌面，刮之难去，或刮之舌面仍有苔迹，舌苔像从舌体长出来的，称为有根苔，属真苔（图3-40）

【临床意义】 判断疾病的轻重与预后。

【机理分析】 真苔是胃气上蒸胃阴，或湿邪、食浊上泛而成，苔有根基，故舌苔与舌体不可分离。疾病的初、中期，舌见真苔，是胃气壅滞、病较深重；病之后期见真苔，为胃气尚存。

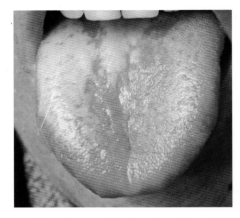

图 3-39 舌色红，舌苔布于舌面右侧，苔黄腻
（男 矽肺伴感染）
A red tongue, and a greasy yellow coating that is distributed on the right side of tongue surface
（male, pneumoconiosis with an infection）

（二）假苔

【舌象特征】 苔不着实，似浮涂舌上，刮之即去，不像是从舌上长出来的，称为无根苔（图3-41）。

【临床意义】 主久病、重病。

【机理分析】 假苔是胃气匮乏，不能续生新苔，而已生之旧苔逐渐脱离舌体，浮于舌面，苔无根基，刮之即去。

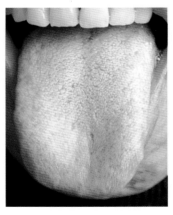

图 3-40 舌色淡红，舌苔白糙紧贴舌面
（女 慢性肾小球肾炎）
A light red tongue, and a white and coarse tongue coating that is closely attached to the tongue surface
（female, chronic glomerular nephritis）

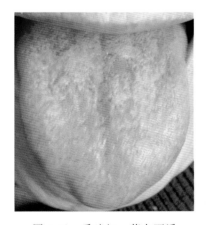

图 3-41 舌暗红，苔白而浮
（女 冠状动脉粥样硬化性心脏病）
A dull red tongue, and a floating white coating
（female, coronary artherosclerotic heart disease）

6. True or False Coating

A tongue coating with or without root is the standard to determine whether a tongue coating is true or false. Generally it is divided into two types: true coating and false coating.

6.1   True Coating

Characteristics: The true tongue coating is closely attached to the surface of the tongue and cannot be easily scraped or wiped off and when scraped, traces of coating remain on the surface of the tongue. The coating appears as if it grows out of the tongue body, hence it is known as coating with root (Diagram 3-40).

Clinical significance: To diagnose the severity of a disease and to determine its prognosis.

Pathogenesis Analysis: The formation of a true tongue coating is by Stomach Qi evaporating the Stomach Yin, or a damp pathogenic factor, or turbid food stagnation upwards to the tongue. The coating has a foundation, thus the tongue coating and tongue body cannot be separated. If a true tongue coating is seen during the initial or intermediate stages of a disease, it indicates that the accumulation and stagnation of Stomach Qi, and the disease is relatively severe; if a true coating is seen during the advanced stages of a disease, it indicates the survival of Stomach Qi.

6.2   False Coating

Characteristics: A coating that does not appear real, seems to be floating or spread onto the tongue, that can be easily wiped or scraped off, and does not grow out of the tongue is known as a false coating or coating without root (Diagram 3-41).

Clinical significance: Indicates chronic disease, severe disease.

Pathogenesis Analysis: A false coating indicates the exhaustion of Stomach Qi, thus failing to produce a new coating, while the existing and old coating is gradually separating from the tongue body, floating on the surface of the tongue. The coating does not have a foundation, so it can be easily scraped off.

第二节 苔 色

苔色的变化主要 有白苔、黄苔、灰黑苔 3 类，临床上可单独出现，也可相兼出现。各种苔色变化需要同苔质、舌色、舌的形态变化结合起来，作具体分析。

一、白苔

白苔是指舌面上的舌苔呈现白色，是最常见的苔色。白苔有厚薄、润燥、腐腻之分。一般分为薄白苔、薄白而润苔、薄白而干苔、薄白而滑苔、白厚腻苔、白厚燥裂苔、白如积粉苔等。

（一）薄白苔

【舌象特征】 舌上薄薄地分布一层白色舌苔，透过舌苔可以看到舌体者，称为薄白苔（图 3-42）。

【临床意义】 可为正常舌苔，疾病情况下主表证，或里证初起。

【机理分析】 薄白苔是临床常见舌苔，可见于外感表证初起。薄白苔亦为正常舌苔的表现之一。

（二）薄白而润苔

【舌象特征】 舌苔薄白而润（图 3-43）。

【临床意义】 为正常舌象；主里证病轻、里证初起、阳虚内寒。

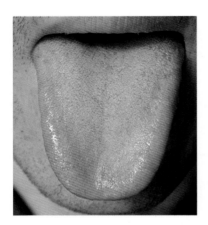

图 3-42 舌色红，苔薄白
（男 左上肢骨折）

A red tongue, and a thin white coating
(male, fracture of the upper left limb)

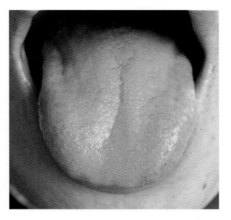

图 3-43 舌色淡红，舌边有瘀点，苔薄白而润
（男 过敏性哮喘急性发作）

A light red tongue, with ecchymoses on the
tongue borders, and a thin white and moist coating
(male, acute attack of allergic asthma)

SECTION TWO   TONGUE COATING COLOR

The different colors of the tongue coating include three types: white coating, yellow coating, and grayish black coating. In clinic, they can appear individually or simultaneously. Inspection of the coating colors should be done together with the examination of changes of the coating proper, tongue body color, tongue body shape to achieve a complete analysis.

1. White Coating

The coating on the surface of the tongue is white in color. It is the most frequently seen coating color and can be a thick or thin coating, moist or dry coating and curdy or greasy coating. It is generally divided as thin white coating, thin white and moist coating, thin white and dry coating, thin white and slippery coating, thick white and greasy coating, thick white and dry coating, and powder-like white coating etc.

1. 1   Thin White Coating

Characteristics: A layer of white coating uniformly and thinly distributed over the surface of the tongue where the tongue body is visible under the coating is known as a thin white coating (Diagram 3-42).

Clinical significance: This is a normal tongue coating, or under pathological conditions, it can indicate an exogenous syndrome, or the initial stage of an interior syndrome.

Pathogenesis Analysis: The thin white coating is the most commonly seen in the clinic, it can appear in the onset of an exogenous syndrome. A thin white tongue coating is also one of the manifestations of a normal tongue coating.

1. 2   Thin, White and Moist Coating

Characteristics: The tongue coating is thin, white, and moist (Diagram 3-43).

Clinical significance: It is the normal manifestation of tongue coating; it can indicate a mild endogenous syndrome, initial stage of an endogenous syndrome, or Yang deficiency with endogenous cold.

【机理分析】 舌苔薄白而润，可为正常舌象，或表证初起，外感邪气尚未入里，舌苔无明显变化，或是里证病轻，或是阳虚内寒，津液未伤，舌苔仍润而薄白。

（三）薄白而滑苔

【舌象特征】 舌苔薄白而滑（图3-44）。
【临床意义】 为外感寒湿，或脾阳不振，水湿内停。
【机理分析】 薄白而滑，多为外感寒湿，水湿上泛于舌面，故苔白而滑。

（四）薄白而干苔

【舌象特征】 舌苔薄白而干（图3-45）。
【临床意义】 见于风热表证。
【机理分析】 风热表证初起，邪热不盛，故苔仍薄白，邪热伤津，故苔干。

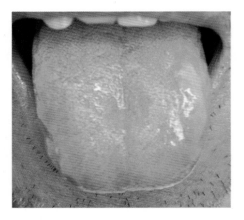

图3-44 舌色暗，苔色白而水滑
（男 2型糖尿病）

A dull tongue, and a watery and slippery
white coating (male, type Ⅱ diabetes)

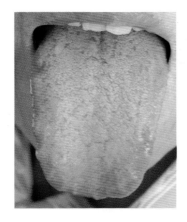

图3-45 舌色暗红，苔白而干（女 冠状
动脉粥样硬化性心脏病，伴上呼吸道感染）

A dull red tongue, and a dry white coating
(female, coronary artherosclerotic heart
disease, upper respiratory tract infection)

（五）白而厚腻苔

【舌象特征】 舌苔白而厚腻（图3-46）。
【临床意义】 湿浊、痰饮、食积。
【机理分析】 苔色白多主表证、寒证。湿浊痰饮为阴邪，湿浊内蕴，阳气被遏，湿浊痰饮食积诸邪上泛于舌面，则苔白而厚腻。

（六）白厚燥裂苔

【舌象特征】 舌苔白厚而燥裂（图3-47）。

Pathogenesis Analysis: A thin, white and moist coating can be a normal manifestation, or indicate the onset of an exogenous syndrome, where the externally contracted pathogenic factor has yet to invade the interior, and there is no evident change to the tongue coating, or it can signify a mild endogenous syndrome, or Yang deficiency with endogenous cold, body fluids are not consumed by pathogenic heat, so the tongue coating is moist, thin and white.

1.3　Thin White and Slippery Coating

Characteristics: The tongue coating is thin, white and slippery (Diagram 3-44).

Clinical significance: It indicates externally contracted damp cold, or depression of Spleen Yang, internal retention of water, and dampness.

Pathogenesis Analysis: Thin, white and slippery coating primarily indicates externally contracted damp cold, water and dampness floods to the tongue surface causing white and slippery coating.

1.4　Thin White and Dry Coating

Characteristics: The tongue coating is thin, white and dry (Diagram 3-45).

Clinical significance: It indicates an exogenous wind heat syndrome.

Pathogenesis Analysis: Thin, white and dry coating is frequently seen in the initial stages of an exogenous wind heat syndrome. Pathogenic heat is not exuberant, thus coating is still thin and white, pathogenic heat has injured fluids, thus the coating is dry.

1.5　White, Thick and Greasy Coating

Characteristics: The tongue coating is white, thick and greasy (Diagram 3-46).

Clinical significance: Indicates damp turbidity, retention of phlegm fluid, or food stagnation.

Pathogenesis Analysis: A white coating generally indicates an exogenous syndrome, cold syndrome. Damp turbidity and phlegm rheum belong to Yin evils. The internal accumulation of damp turbidity leads to the obstruction of Yang Qi. Damp turbidity, phlegm rheum, food stagnation all flood upwards to the surface of the tongue, causing a white, thick and greasy coating.

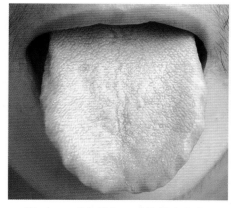

图 3-46　舌色淡红，舌前部有齿痕，
苔厚白而腻（男　扩张型心肌病）
A light red tongue, with teeth-marks on the anterior, and a thick white and greasy coating (male, dilated myocardiopathy)

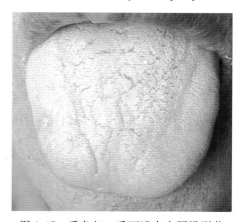

图 3-47　舌色红，舌面满布白厚燥裂苔
（男　慢性阻塞性肺气肿）
A red tongue, and a thick white and dry coating completely covering the tongue surface (male, chronic obstructive pulmonary emphysema)

1.6　Thick, White and Dry Coating.

Characteristics: The tongue coating is white, thick and dry (Diagram 3-47).

【临床意义】 主燥热伤津。

【机理分析】 白厚而燥裂多为邪热耗伤津液。

（七）白如积粉苔

【舌象特征】 苔白如积粉，扪之不燥者，为积粉苔（图3-48）。

【临床意义】 常见于外感温疫和内痈。

【机理分析】 积粉苔是由外感秽浊不正之气与热毒相结而成。

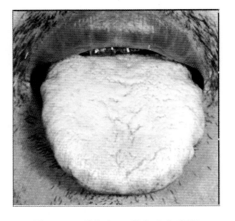

图 3-48　舌色红，苔色白如积粉
（男　艾滋病）
A red tongue, and a white powder-like
coating (male, AIDS)

二、黄苔

舌苔呈现黄色谓之黄苔。根据黄色的浅深，黄苔有淡黄、深黄和焦黄苔之别；黄苔可与白苔同见，而见黄白相间苔；黄苔还有厚薄、润燥、腐腻等苔质变化，而见薄黄苔、黄厚苔、黄腻苔、黄滑苔。

（一）淡黄苔

【舌象特征】 淡黄苔又称微黄苔，是在薄白苔上出现均匀的浅黄色，多由薄白苔转化而成（图3-49）。

【临床意义】 主热证、里证之轻证。

【机理分析】 由于热邪熏灼，故苔现黄色。

（二）深黄苔

【舌象特征】 深黄苔又称正黄苔，苔色黄而略深厚（图3-50）。

【临床意义】 深黄苔主里热深重。

【机理分析】 邪热上熏于舌面，故苔色见黄。苔色愈黄，邪热愈甚。深黄苔为热重。

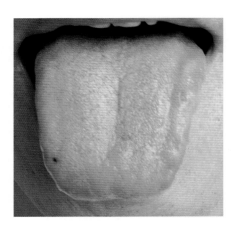

图 3-49　舌色红，舌苔淡黄而薄
（男　2型糖尿病）
A red tongue, and a thin pale yellow
tongue coating (male, type II diabetes)

Clinical significance: Indicating evile heat consuming the body fluids.

Pathogenesis Analysis: A coating that is thick, white and dry is primarily the manifestation of body fluids consumed by the evile heat.

1. 7　White Powder-like Coating

Characteristics: A white coating that appears powder-like and on palpation does not feel dry is a white powder-like coating (Diagram 3-48).

Clinical significance: Often seen in externally contracted pestilence and internal abscesses.

Pathogenesis Analysis: Its formation is due to the intermingling of an externally contracted filthy, turbid evil and heat toxin.

2. Yellow Coating

A yellow coating refers to a tongue coating that appears yellow in color. According to the intensity of the yellow color, there are pale yellow coating, dark yellow coating, and sallow yellow coating. A yellow coating can be seen together with a white coating, appearing as the interspersing of yellow and white colored coating. A yellow coating can also be either thick or thin, moist or dry, curdy or greasy etc. Thus there are thin yellow coating, thick yellow coating, greasy yellow coating, or slippery yellow coating.

2. 1　Pale Yellow Coating

Characteristics: A pale yellow coating also known as a slight yellow coating is similar to a thin white coating except that there is an even distribution of a pale yellow color, and it is usually transformed from a pale white coating (Diagram 3-49).

Clinical significance: It indicates heat syndrome and a mild interior syndrome.

Pathogenesis Analysis: The nature of pathogenic heat is to burn and scorch, thus the coating appears yellow.

2. 2　Deep Yellow Coating

Characteristics: Deep yellow coating is also known as proper yellow coating. The coating is a solid yellow color (Diagram 3-50).

Clinical significance: Signifies severe internal heat.

Pathogenesis Analysis: Pathogenic heat smokes upwards to the surface of the tongue, thus causing the coating to become yellow. The deeper the yellow, the stronger the pathogenic heat, thus a deep yellow coating indicates severe heat.

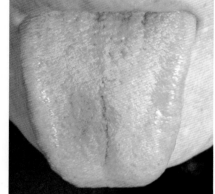

图 3-50　舌色红，舌苔深黄而厚腐
（男　慢性浅表性胃炎）
A red tongue, and a thick deep yellow and curdy tongue coating (male, chronic superficial gastritis)

（三）焦黄苔

【舌象特征】 焦黄苔又称老黄苔，是正黄色中夹有灰褐色苔者（图3-51）。

【临床意义】 主里热极盛。

【机理分析】 焦黄苔为邪热伤津，燥结腑实之证。

（四）黄白相间苔

【舌象特征】 舌苔由白转黄或黄白相间（图3-52）。

【临床意义】 为外感表证、表里相兼、表邪入里化热的阶段。

【机理分析】 舌苔由白转黄或黄白相间为外感表证、表里相兼、表邪入里化热的阶段。故《伤寒指掌·察舌辨症法》说："但看舌苔带一分白，病亦带一分表，必纯黄无白，邪方离表入里。"

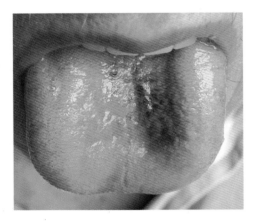

图3-51 舌色红，舌体肿胀，舌苔黄中带黑
（男 冠心病 心房颤动）
A red and swollen tongue, and a yellow black tongue coating (male, coronary heart disease, atrial fibrillation)

（五）薄黄苔

【舌象特征】 舌苔薄黄（图3-53）。

【临床意义】 见于风热表证，或风寒化热入里，邪热未甚。

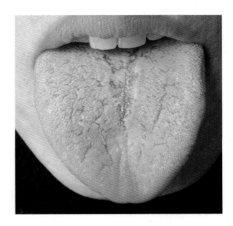

图3-52 舌色红，舌苔黄白相间，苔中裂
（男 急性上呼吸道感染）
A red tongue, with a yellow and white tongue coating, and a fissure in the centre of the coating (male, acute upper respiratory tract infection)

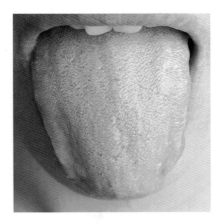

图3-53 舌色淡红，苔薄黄
（女 2型糖尿病）
A light red tongue, and a thin yellow coating (female, type Ⅱ diabetes)

2. 3 Sallow Coating

Characteristics: A sallow coating is also known as an aged yellow coating. It is a proper yellow coating mixed with a grayish hue in the coating (Diagram 3-51).

Clinical significance: It indicates extreme exuberance of internal heat.

Pathogenesis Analysis: Being the consumption of fluids by pathogenic heat, leading to the retention of dryness and an excess of the Fu syndrome.

2. 4 Yellow and White Coating

Characteristics: It is the transformation of a white coating to a yellow coating or white and yellow coating occurring simultaneously (Diagram 3-52).

Clinical significance: It indicates an externally contracted superficial syndrome, or a dual interior exterior syndrome, or the process of exogenous pathogenic factor invading the interior and transforming heat.

Pathogenesis Analysis: The tongue coating is due to the transformation of a white coating to a yellow coating or white and yellow coating indicating an externally contracted superficial syndrome, or a dual interior exterior syndrome, or the process of exogenous pathogenic factor invading the interior and transforming heat, thus *Grasping Cold-induced Diseases · Method for Differentiating Syndromes by Observing the Tongue* states: "To see a tongue coating that bears a bit of white indicates that a part of the disease is in the exterior. If the coating is purely yellow, it indicates the pathogenic factor has left the exterior and invaded the interior. "

2. 5 Thin Yellow Coating

Characteristics: The tongue coating is thin and yellow (Diagram 3-53).

Clinical significance: It is seen in an exogenous wind heat syndrome, or when wind cold transforms into heat and invades the interior, pathogenic heat is still mild.

【机理分析】 薄黄苔示在疾病过程中见之，主邪气不盛，黄苔主邪热上熏，故薄黄苔主邪热未盛。

（六）黄厚苔

【舌象特征】 舌苔黄厚（图 3-54，3-55）。

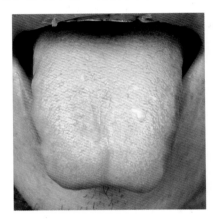 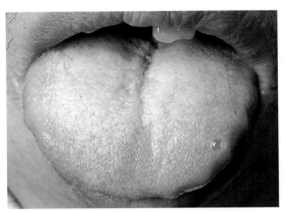

图 3-54　舌色淡红，边有齿痕，舌苔淡黄滑　　　　图 3-55　舌色红，苔淡黄厚腻
（男　慢性浅表性胃炎）　　　　　　　　　　　　（男　慢性浅表性胃炎）

A light red tongue, with tooth-marked borders,　　A red tongue, and a pale yellow, thick and greasy
and a pale yellow and slippery tongue coating　　　　coating (male, chronic superficial gastritis)
（male, chronic superficial gastritis)

【临床意义】 见于里实热证。
【机理分析】 里热炽盛，熏蒸于上，故苔黄厚。

（七）黄滑苔

【舌象特征】 舌淡胖嫩，苔淡黄而润滑多津（图 3-56）。
【临床意义】 主湿热之邪。
【机理分析】 多为阳虚寒湿之体，痰饮聚而化热；或是气血亏虚者，感受湿热之邪所致。

（八）黄腻苔

【舌象特征】 舌苔黄而苔质腻者（图 3-57，3-58）。
【临床意义】 湿热、痰饮，或食积等证，为湿热蕴结之象。
【机理分析】 湿盛上泛于舌面则苔腻，热盛则苔色黄。

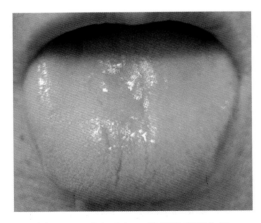

图 3-56　舌色暗红，舌苔淡黄而水滑
（女　乏力待查）

A dull red tongue, and a watery and slippery pale yellow
tongue coating (female, lassitude awaiting examination)

Pathogenesis Analysis: A thin yellow coating seen during the course of a disease indicates pathogenic factor is still mild, and yellow coating indicates upward smoking of pathogenic heat, so a thin yellow coating indicates pathogenic heat has not yet to become exuberant.

2.6 Thick Yellow Coating

Characteristics: Tongue coating is thick and yellow (Diagram 3-54, 3-55).

Clinical significance: It is seen in endogenous excess heat syndrome.

Pathogenesis Analysis: Interior scorching of exuberant heat fumigating upwards thus a thick yellow coating results.

2.7 Yellow and Slippery Coating

Characteristics: Tongue body is pale, enlarged and tender. The coating is pale yellow, slippery with copious fluids (Diagram 3-56).

Clinical significance: Suggests a damp heat pathogen.

Pathogenesis Analysis: Predominantly seen in individuals that has Yang deficiency with damp cold, accumulating of phlegm fluid and transforming to heat; or individuals who has Qi and Blood deficiency resulting from an exogenous damp heat pathogen.

2.8 Yellow Greasy Coating

Characteristics: The tongue coating is a yellow color and its texture is greasy (Diagram 3-57, 3-58).

Clinical significance: Indicates syndromes of damp heat, retention of phlegm fluid, or food stagnation etc, being the manifestation of the accumulation of damp heat.

Pathogenesis Analysis: The exuberance of damp floods to the tongue surface causing a greasy coating, and the exuberance of heat results in a yellow coating.

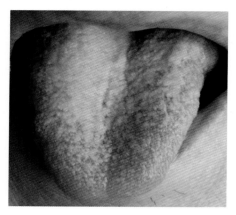

图 3-57 舌色红，舌苔淡黄厚腻
（男　冠心病、心律失常）

A red tongue, and pale yellow, thick and greasy tongue coating (male, coronary heart disease, arrhythmia)

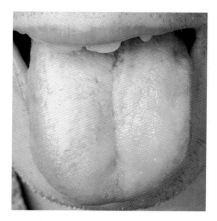

图 3-58 舌色暗红，舌苔前部少苔，中根部黄厚腻
（男　黄疸待查）

A dull red tongue, with scanty coating at the anterior, and a thick, greasy and yellow coating at the centre and root (male, jaundice awaiting examination)

三、灰黑苔

【舌象特征】 灰苔与黑苔同类，苔色浅黑为灰苔，苔色深黑为黑苔，并称为灰黑苔（图3-59）。

【临床意义】 主邪热炽盛，或阴寒内盛、痰湿久郁等证。

【机理分析】 苔色浅深与疾病性质相应。一般说黑苔多在疾病持续一定时日，发展到相当程度后才出现。灰黑苔既可见于里热证，也可见于里寒证，但无论寒热均属重证。灰黑色浅而润多主寒，色深而燥多属热。黑色越深病情越重。

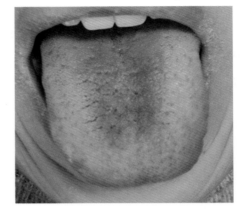

图3-59 舌色紫暗，舌苔焦黄灰黑而厚
（女 原发性肝癌）
A dull purple tongue, and a sallow yellow-black and thick tongue coating (female, primary Liver cancer)

苔质润燥是鉴别黑苔寒热属性的又一重要指征。若舌苔灰黑湿润多津是寒湿内蕴，多由白苔转化而来，常见于寒湿为病；而灰黑舌苔干燥无津，多由黄苔转变而来，属热盛伤津，常见于热性病中，也可见于阴虚火旺。

灰黑苔根据苔色的浅深及润燥一般分为灰黑湿润苔、白腻灰黑苔、黄腻灰黑苔、焦黑干燥苔。

（一）灰黑湿润苔

【舌象特征】 舌苔灰黑湿润多津（图3-60，3-61）。

【临床意义】 多由白苔转化而来，常见于寒湿为病。

【机理分析】 多属阳虚寒湿、痰饮内停，则见苔湿润，色灰黑。

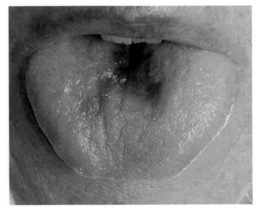

图3-60 舌淡红，舌苔灰黑而厚腻
（男 骨髓增生异常综合征、Ⅰ型糖尿病）
A light red tongue, and a grayish black, thick and greasy tongue coating (male, myelodysplastic syndrome, type Ⅰ diabetes)

3. Grayish Black Coating

Characteristics: A gray coating and black coating are of the same type. A pale black coating is also a gray coating, and a deep black coating is simply a black coating (Diagram 3-59).

Clinical significance: It indicates syndromes of exuberant heat pathogen, or exuberant Yin and cold, chronic stagnation of phlegm dampness.

Pathogenesis Analysis: The paleness or darkness of a coating color corresponds to the nature of a disease. Generally speaking, a black coating appears when the disease is of long duration and developed to a certain degree. A grayish black coating can be seen in an endogenous heat syndrome or endogenous cold syndrome. Whether it is a heat syndrome or cold syndrome, it suggests a severe syndrome. A pale grayish black and moist coating mainly indicates a cold syndrome, while a deep grayish black and dry coating primarily indicates a heat syndrome. The darker the black color, the more severe the disease.

Determining the moisture of a black coating is important to differentiate the heat or cold nature. If a grayish black tongue coating is moist with copious fluids, it indicates interior retention of damp cold, predominantly evolved from a white coating caused by damp cold; a grayish black and dry coating with absence of fluids is primarily evolved from a yellow coating, where exuberant heat has consumed the body fluids, mainly due to a febrile natured disease, or Yin deficiency with up-flaming of fire.

A grayish black coating is generally subdivided according to the intensity of the coating color and its moisture. There are grayish black and moist coating, white greasy grayish black coating, yellow greasy and grayish black coating, and scorched black and dry coating.

3.1   Grayish Black and Moist Coating

Characteristics: Tongue coating is grayish black in color and moist with copious fluids (Diagram 3-60, 3-61).

Clinical significance: Mainly evolved from a white coating, seen in damp cold syndromes.

Pathogenesis Analysis: Primarily indicative of Yang deficiency and damp cold, internal retention of phlegm rheum results in a moist coating that is grayish black in color.

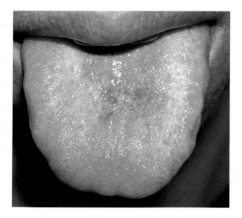

图 3-61   舌色红，舌苔中灰褐而厚腻
（男   冠状动脉粥样硬化性心脏病）

A red tongue, and a grayish brown, thick and greasy tongue coating (male, coronary artherosclerotic heart disease)

（二）白腻灰黑苔

【舌象特征】 苔白腻灰黑，舌面湿润，舌质淡白胖嫩（图3-62）。

【临床意义】 主寒证、痰湿久郁等证。

【机理分析】 寒湿内蕴，积久而成。

（三）黄腻灰黑苔

【舌象特征】 舌苔黄腻灰黑（图3-63）。

【临床意义】 湿热内停证。

【机理分析】 黄腻灰黑苔多为湿热内蕴，日久不化所致。

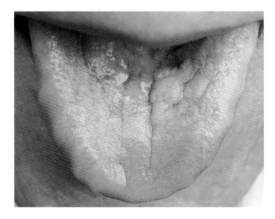

图 3-62 舌色红，边有齿痕，舌苔灰黑而腻
（男 高血压病）

A red tongue, tooth-marked borders, and a greasy
grayish black tongue coating (male, hypertension)

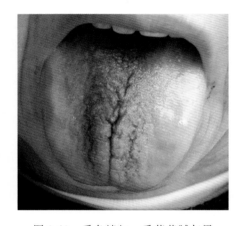

图 3-63 舌色淡红，舌苔黄腻灰黑
（女 胃癌）

A light red tongue, and a greasy, yellow, grayish
black tongue coating (female, Stomach cancer)

（四）焦黑干燥苔

【舌象特征】 苔焦黑干燥，舌质干裂起刺（图3-64）。

【临床意义】 热极津枯之证。

【机理分析】 苔焦黑干燥，舌质干裂起刺者，不论病起外感或内伤，均为热极津枯之证。

In an externally contracted disease, a thin coating that changes to a thick one suggests the pathogenic factor in the exterior has invaded the interior; a white coating that turns yellow is a sign that the pathogenic factor has transformed to heat; tongue color that turns red and tongue coating that is dry indicates the exuberance of pathogenic heat, and the blazing of both Qi and nutrient; a peeled tongue coating and deep red tongue proper is seen when heat has entered the nutritive and Blood levels, consumption of both Qi and Yin etc. During the course of development of an internal impairment and miscellaneous disease, the manifestations of the tongue follow a set pattern in their changes. For instance, wind-stroke patients have light red tongues and coatings that are thin and white, suggesting the mildness of the disease, a favorable prognosis. When the tongue changes from light red to red, dull red, deep red, or a dull purple color, tongue coating to yellow and greasy, or scorched black, or the vessels under the tongue are swollen, this indicates wind phlegm transformed to heat and blood stasis. On the other hand, when a tongue color changes from a dull red or dull purple to a light red color, and gradual change of the tongue coating, it mainly indicates the favorable turn of the disease. Understanding the relation between the tongue manifestations and the developmental changes of a disease can adequately assist in the identification of the pathological changes that occur at different stages of a disease, laying the basis for an early diagnosis and hence prompt treatment.

SECTION TWO   THE CLINICAL SIGNIFICANCE
OF TONGUE DIAGNOSIS

The tongue manifestations can be a relatively objective reflection on the state of a disease. Therefore, its significance is crucial to the clinical differentiation of syndromes, establishing treatment method, the use of formulas and herbs, judging the progress of the disease, and the analysis of its prognosis. As the *Methods for Examination of the Tongue in Practice • Treatise on Tongue Examination as the Overall Standard for Observing Symptoms* states: "For all internal and external miscellaneous diseases, there isn't one that does not have a form on the tongue, whose Qi is marked on the tongue, ···relying on the tongue to distinguish between deficiency and excess. If it is not clear, then depend on the tongue to distinguish between Yin and Yang, and if Yin and Yang are clearly defined then use the tongue to distinguish the internal organs involved, and to choose a formula, and thereafter if there is no worsening of the internal organs, then there is no error in the formula. During a time of urgency and difficulty, where there are no signs to consult, and pulses cannot be felt, there is still the tongue to be relied upon; in gynecological and pediatric diseases, where the examination methods of smelling and hearing come to no avail, and asking is futile, the tongue is the only method to be relied upon." The clinical significances are:

一、判断邪正盛衰

正气的盛衰能明显地在舌上反映出来，如气血充盛则舌色淡红而润；气血不足则舌色淡白。气滞血瘀则舌色青紫或舌下络脉怒张。津液充足则舌质舌苔滋润；津液不足则舌干苔燥。胃气旺盛则舌苔有根；胃气衰败则舌苔无根或光剥无苔。脏腑功能失常亦常见于舌，如脾失健运，湿邪困阻每见舌苔厚腻；肝风内动多有舌体震颤或歪斜；心脾郁热，则舌生疮疡、红肿热痛或吐舌、弄舌等。

二、区别病邪性质

不同的病邪致病，舌象特征亦各异。如外感风寒，苔多薄白，外感风热，苔多薄黄，说明感邪性质不同，舌象的表现也不同。寒湿为病，舌淡而苔白滑；痰饮、湿浊、食滞或外感秽浊之气，均可见舌苔厚腻；燥热为病，则舌红苔燥；瘀血内阻，舌紫暗或有瘀点等。故风、寒、热、燥、湿、痰、瘀、食等诸种病因，大多可从舌象上加以辨别。

三、分析病位浅深

病邪轻、浅多见舌苔变化，而病情深、重可见舌苔舌质同时变化。以外感温热病而言，其病位可划分为卫、气、营、血4个层次。邪在卫分，可见舌苔薄白；邪入气分，舌苔白厚而干或见黄苔，舌色红；舌绛可见于邪入营分；舌色深红、紫绛或紫暗，舌枯少苔或无苔为邪入血分。说明不同的舌象提示病位浅深不同。

1. Judging the Sufficiency or Insufficiency of the Anti-pathogenic Qi and the Pathogenic Factor

The tongue can clearly reflect the state of the anti-pathogenic Qi. If Qi and Blood is prosperous in the body, the tongue color will be light red and moist; if Qi and Blood are insufficient the tongue color is pale white. The stagnation of Qi and Blood results in cyanosis of the tongue or the swelling of the vessels under the tongue. When the body fluids are flourished, the tongue proper and tongue coating are nourished and moist. If the body fluids are deficient then both the tongue body and tongue coating become dry. When Stomach Qi is prospering, the tongue coating has root; yet when Stomach Qi has deteriorated, then the tongue coating is without root or a tongue that is shiny and bald without coating. Dysfunctions of the internal organs can also be seen on the tongue. For example, when there is a dysfunction of the Spleen in transportation, pathogenic damp obstructs, resulting in a thick and greasy tongue coating; the internal stirring of Liver wind sees quivering or deviation of the tongue body; in stagnation of heat in the Heart and Spleen, ulcers are formed on the tongue, which becomes red, swollen and has a burning pain. Sometimes, a protruding or wagging tongue develops.

2. Distinguishing the Nature of the Pathogenic Factor

In accordance with the different pathogenic factors that cause disease, the changes in manifestations on the tongue correspond accordingly. For instance, with exogenous wind cold the coating is mostly thin and white; with exogenous wind heat the coating is usually thin and yellow; It shows that the difference in pathogenic factors results in different manifestations of the tongue. In a damp cold syndrome, the tongue is pale and the coating is white and slippery; phlegm fluid retention, damp turbidity, and food stagnation or an exogenous filthy and turbid Qi can all result in a thick and greasy tongue coating; a dry heat syndrome sees a red tongue and dry coating; internal obstruction of blood stasis results in cyanosis of the tongue that can have purple spots etc. Thus wind, cold, heat, dry, damp, phlegm, blood stasis, food etc can all be the cause of disease, and most of them can be further differentiated based on the tongue manifestations.

3. Analyzing the Location and Depth of Disease

A pathogenic factor that is mild and shallow (in the exterior) mainly sees changes in the tongue coating while a disease that is deep (in the interior) and severe can see changes in both the tongue body and tongue coating. Such as exogenous febrile diseases, the location of disease can be assigned to 4 levels, the defense level, the Qi level, the nutritive level, and the Blood level. A pathogenic factor in the defense level sees a thin white tongue coating; a pathogen that has entered the Qi level can result in a thick white and dry tongue coating or a red tongue with yellow coating; a tongue that is crimson the pathogen has entered the nutritive level; a deep red, purplish and deep red, or dull purple, withered tongue with scanty coating or no coating indicates the pathogen has entered the Blood level. It signifies that different manifestations of the tongue can identify the location and depth of disease.

四、推断病势进退

病情发展的进退趋势，可从舌象上反映出来。由此，可以推断病势的变化情况。从舌苔上看，舌苔由白转黄，由黄转焦黑色，苔质由润转燥，提示热邪由轻变重、由表及里，津液耗损；反之，苔由厚变薄，由黄转白，由燥变润，为邪热渐退，津液复生，病情向好的趋势转变。若舌苔突然剥落，舌面光滑无苔，是邪盛正衰，胃气、胃阴暴绝的证候；薄苔突然增厚，是病邪急剧入里的表现，两者均为恶候。从舌质观察，舌色淡红转红、绛，甚至转为绛紫，或舌上起刺，是邪热深入营血，有伤阴、血瘀之势；舌色由淡红转为淡白、淡青紫，或舌胖嫩湿润，则为阳气受伤，阴寒渐盛，病邪由表入里，由轻转重，由单纯变复杂，病势在进展。

五、估计病情预后

舌荣有神，舌面有苔，舌态正常者为邪气未盛，正气未伤之象，预后较好。舌质枯晦，舌苔无根，舌态异常者为正气亏损，胃气衰败，病情多凶险。

4. Inferring the Progress and Momentum of Disease

The tongue can also reflect the progress of a disease in its tendency to advance or retreat. From this it is possible to deduce the condition of changes in the momentum of a disease. From observing the tongue coating, a coating that changes from white to yellow, from yellow to a scorched black color, the coating proper from moist to dry, it indicates that pathogenic heat has transformed from mild to severe, from just the exterior to the interior, and the consumption of fluids; alternatively a coating that changes from thick to thin, from yellow to white, from dry to moist, indicates pathogenic heat is gradually retreating, the recovering production of body fluids, and the tendency of the disease is taking a favorable turn. If a tongue coating suddenly peels off leaving a shiny and slippery tongue surface without coating, it indicates exuberance of the pathogenic factor and the decline of the anti-pathogenic Qi, the sudden collapse of Stomach Yin and Stomach Qi; the sudden change of a tongue coating from thin to thick specifies the rapid invasion of the pathogen into the interior, the two being vicious manifestations. From observation of the tongue proper, a light red tongue changing to a red, deep red, or even a purplish deep red color, or prickles appearing on the tongue signifies that the momentum of pathogenic heat has invaded deep into the nutritive and Blood levels and consumed Yin and stagnated Blood; a light red tongue that changes to a pale white, or pale cyanosis of the tongue, or to an enlarged, tender and moist tongue indicates injury to Yang Qi, the gradual exuberance of Yin cold, the pathogen transferring from the exterior to the interior, from mild to severe, from simple to complicated, shows that the disease is advancing.

5. Predicting the Prognosis of a Disease

The mark of a favorable prognosis includes a flourishing tongue with spirit, a coating on the tongue surface, and normal movement of the tongue indicating that the pathogenic factor has not yet to prosper and the anti-pathogenic Qi has not waned. A withered and dull tongue proper, a coating without root and abnormal movement of the tongue suggests the decline of anti-pathogenic Qi, the deterioration of Stomach Qi, and an unfavorable and dangerous prognosis.